The Ultimate Guide to Weight-Loss Surgery

Mr. Roger Ackroyd | Miss Corinne Owers

Dr. Chinnadorai Rajeswaran | Mrs. Nerissa Walker

Copyright © 2014 Ackroyd, Owers, Rajeswaran, Walker

All rights reserved.

ISBN-13: 978-1496010315
ISBN-10: 1496010310

For many people, weight-loss diets can be a difficult and time-consuming pre-occupation, with often disappointing, short-term weight-loss results. For some people, bariatric (weight loss) surgery is an effective long-term tool to aid weight loss and gain control over their eating, weight and health.

However, for those people considering or already on their weight-loss surgery journey, the information and advice available for weight-loss surgery can often be conflicting, inconsistent, confusing, and unreliable.

The **simply***bariatrics* The Ultimate Guide to Weight-Loss Surgery has been written to provide reliable information for people who are considering weight-loss surgery, having surgery, or going through lifelong maintenance. It will provide all the information, practical tips, and tools you will ever need.

Written by well-recognised weight-loss surgery medical professionals, this book brings together expert advice and practical information making it the most comprehensive reference book available for people before and after weight-loss surgery.

You will find this a very comprehensive, easy-to-read book that is both informative and easy to use, supporting you all the way through your weight-loss journey.

Mr. Roger Ackroyd
Consultant Bariatric Surgeon
MBChB, MD(Dist), FRCS, FRCS(Ed), FRCS (Gen Surg)
Director of **simply***bariatrics*

Dr. Chinnadorai Rajeswaran ("Dr. Raj")
Consultant Physician, Obesity, Diabetes and Endocrinology
MBBS, FRCP, MSc
Director of **simply***bariatrics*

Miss Corinne Owers
Specialist Registrar in General Surgery and Clinical Research Fellow
MBChB, MRCS, PGDipMedEd

Mrs. Nerissa Walker
Registered Specialist Dietitian for Obesity and Bariatric surgery
BSc (Hons), RD, PG.Dip. HCPC

TABLE OF CONTENTS

FOREWORD I

WHAT IS OBESITY AND WHAT DOES IT MEAN FOR ME? 1
    WHAT PROBLEMS CAN OBESITY CAUSE? 3
    PHYSICAL HEALTH PROBLEMS 5
    SHOULD I SEEK HELP FOR MY WEIGHT? 11

DIETS AND CONSEQUENCES OF DIETING 13
    CAN MEDICALLY UNSUPERVISED DIETS MAKE YOU OBESE? 15
    OTHER WEIGHT LOSS STRATEGIES 16

AM I SUITABLE FOR WEIGHT-LOSS (BARIATRIC) SURGERY?
.... 20
    GUIDELINES FOR WEIGHT-LOSS SURGERY 22
    GOVERNMENT (STATE) FUNDED BARIATRIC SURGERY 24
    BARIATRIC SURGERY IN PRIVATE HOSPITALS (SELF-FUNDED) 26
    WHEN IS WEIGHT-LOSS SURGERY NOT RECOMMENDED? 27

DIFFERENT TYPES OF WEIGHT-LOSS SURGERY 30
    COMPARISON OF WEIGHT-LOSS SURGERY OPERATIONS 40

HOW TO ARRANGE BARIATRIC SURGERY 42
    HOW TO CHOOSE A SURGEON 43
    HOW TO CHOOSE A SURGEON IN A PRIVATE SETTING 45
    HOW TO CHOOSE THE RIGHT HOSPITAL 45
    COST OF HAVING WEIGHT-LOSS SURGERY 48
    HEALTH TOURISM FOR WEIGHT-LOSS SURGERY 49
    CHECK LIST FOR HAVING BARIATRIC SURGERY ABROAD: 50

PREPARATION FOR BARIATRIC SURGERY 52
    DISCUSS BARIATRIC SURGERY PLANS WITH FAMILY & FRIENDS 52

- Pre-Surgery Dietary and Lifestyle Changes 53
- Investigations Before Weight-Loss Surgery 56
- Dietary Preparation before Weight-loss surgery 60
- Pre-Operative Liver Shrinkage Diet 61
- Vitamin and Mineral Supplementation 64
- Medication 65
- Childcare and Dependents 65
- Driving 66
- Work 66
- What to Bring into Hospital 67
- Support Groups and Internet Forums 68
- Conclusion 69

WHAT HAPPENS BEFORE, DURING AND AFTER WEIGHT-LOSS SURGERY? 71
- Before Surgery 71
- During the Hospital Stay 72
- After Surgery 75

COMPLICATIONS OR PROBLEMS AFTER WEIGHT-LOSS SURGERY 79
- General Complications 80
- Early Complications 82
- Late Complications 86
- Other Effects of Bariatric Surgery 94
- When to Seek Urgent Help after Weight-Loss Surgery? 96

CARE AND RECOVERY AFTER BARIATRIC SURGERY 98
- Follow-up by the Bariatric Team 98
- Family and Friends 100

PHYSICAL ACTIVITY AFTER BARIATRIC SURGERY 108
- MET for Various Physical Activities 111

EXERCISE PROTOCOL AFTER BARIATRIC SURGERY 114

SEX AND RELATIONSHIPS AFTER BARIATRIC SURGERY ..120
- POST-SURGICAL SEX LIFE 120
- POST-SURGICAL RELATIONSHIPS 123

PRE-CONCEPTION AND PREGNANCY AFTER BARIATRIC SURGERY 130

WEIGHT REGAIN AFTER BARIATRIC SURGERY 142

YOUR RELATIONSHIP WITH FOOD 152
- PREFACE 152
- INTRODUCTION 153
- RELATIONSHIP WITH FOOD 156
- THE RELATIONSHIP WITH FOOD DIARY 157
- GUIDANCE ON COMPLETING THE DIARY 158

FOOD GROUPS: PROTEIN, FAT, AND CARBS.......................170
- PROTEIN 171
- CARBOHYDRATES 174
- FAT..175

RECIPES...178
- STAGE ONE — LIQUIDS ONLY 178
- STAGE ONE RECIPES 181
- STAGE TWO— PUREED 184
- STAGE TWO RECIPES 185
- STAGE THREE—SOFT, MUSHY AND CRISPY 187
- STAGE THREE RECIPES 188
- STAGE FOUR—NORMAL TEXTURED DIET 193
- STAGE FOUR RECIPES 194

TOP TIPS FOR AFTER SURGERY 202
- EATING OUT 202

BUYING NEW CLOTHES 203
COVERING LOOSE SKIN 203
AVOID OVER-EATING 204
FOLLOW UP AND SUPPORT 205
USEFUL LINKS 206

Foreword

Bariatric surgery, or obesity surgery, has been rediscovered in the last 15 years after a shaky start with some procedures that were notorious for long-term complications. In addition, the advent of keyhole surgery in recent decades has made surgery, in general, much more acceptable.

This is especially true for obese people, because it has resulted in a decline in surgical complications and an earlier return to normal activities. There have also been considerable improvements in the procedures available for treating severe obesity. This is all superimposed upon an obesity epidemic that has increased demand for effective treatment for those who are very obese.

Indeed, the main problem now is not what should we do for our severely obese patient but rather how can we deliver enough of our effective surgical treatments to those who need it. There is also a dearth of good up-to-date literature for patients who may be considering a surgical option for their obesity problem to read—a patient who has some knowledge about possible surgical options prior to approaching a bariatric unit is likely to have a better outcome from their surgery.

Whilst the explosion in Internet sites dealing with obesity surgery can be useful, they often suffer from bias and lack of robustness. Research in obesity surgery has now clearly established it as adding life years, reducing long-term problems such as diabetes, and improving the quality of life for those who undertake it. But, like most surgery, there are some risks and complications that the new patient needs to be aware of.

It was a pleasure to review this multi-author book, which achieves its aim to be comprehensive, covering all aspects of bariatric surgery that the potential patient needs to be aware of. The contributors are all highly experienced and pass on their knowledge from many years experience in developing and maintaining a bariatric service in the United Kingdom.

Some units offering bariatric services are not comprehensive in their pre-operative advice and this book goes a long way in raising all the relevant issues that the potential patient needs to be aware of and request answers before they commit themselves to a surgical option for their obesity. Indeed, some bariatric surgeons are likely to suggest that it should be required reading for any potential bariatric patient and they should be tested on understanding its content before they are accepted for surgery. It cannot be understated enough that any potential patient needs to thoroughly understand all aspects of their intended surgical procedure in order to get the best results from the very small risk they are taking in order to benefit from the surgery. This book deals comprehensively with all aspects surrounding the intended surgery, providing information that, in former times, was simply neglected by many surgical teams.

The particular strengths of this book are that it is written in plain language that the new patient can easily understand. Furthermore, it is very up-to-date in current thinking about procedures offered, complications, and all the surrounding issues that concern patients, such as changes in diet and eating behaviour, social aspects, and long-term issues. No doubt the authors will constantly update it as new knowledge becomes available. I recommend this book to all patients who intend to make use of our new knowledge and skills in surgery to treat their obesity problem.

John Baxter
Emeritus Professor of Surgery
Swansea University, UK
Founder and Former President
of the British Obesity
and Metabolic Surgery Society

Chapter 1
What is Obesity and What Does It Mean for Me?

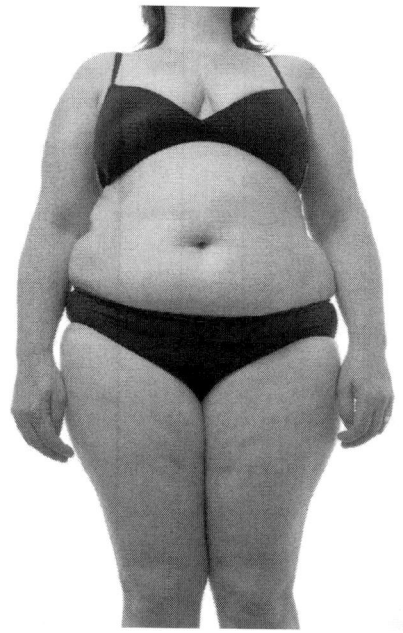

How Do I Know If I Am Obese?

'Obesity' is a medical condition describing people who weigh more than they should. When we talk about obesity, we are referring to the fact that a person's weight is causing them health problems, which they may not have had if they weighed less.

Although there are many different ways of describing a person's size, most healthcare professionals use a tool called the "Body Mass Index" or BMI. We can work out what a person's BMI is by measuring their height (in metres) and weight (in kilograms) and then using the following formula:

$$BMI = Weight / height^2$$

BMI	Classification
Less than 18.5	Underweight
18.5-24.9	Healthy weight
25.0-29.9	Overweight
30.0-34.9	Class 1 obesity
35.0-39.9	Class 2 obesity
Over 40	Class 3 obesity

Once this total has been calculated, the doctor, nurse, or dietitian can see how overweight you are.

If you have a BMI of over 35, you are classed as 'severe obese'.

If you have a BMI of more than 40, or have a BMI of over 35 with obesity related health problems (such as type 2 diabetes, high blood pressure, depression), you are classed as 'morbidly obese'. You may therefore be eligible for weight-loss surgery.

What Problems Can Obesity Cause?

There are many physical and mental health problems, which can be caused by obesity.

Physical health problems include the following:

- High blood pressure
- Heart failure
- Blood clots
- High cholesterol
- Type 2 diabetes (also known as "late onset diabetes")
- Sleep apnoea (interruption to breathing when asleep)
- Arthritis
- Back pain
- Infertility
- Skin problems
- Liver disease
- Certain types of cancer

Obesity puts a lot of strain on your body. The more obese a person is, the more strain there is on the body, and the more likely a person is to have problems.

Obesity is known to shorten a person's life expectancy. On average, a person with obesity lives five to ten years less than someone with a normal weight. The chance of a person with obesity dying early from heart disease or diabetes is much higher than a person who is not obese.

When someone is obese, the tissues in the body become inflamed (like the knee after an injury for example). This inflammation causes damage to organs such as the liver and blood vessels. It also affects the body's immune system, so people get chest, skin, bladder, or wound infections much more easily. In some cases, these infections can become very serious because they are more difficult to treat, and that person may become seriously ill.

Although not everyone with obesity will have major health problems, most will have at least one or two. Research and experience with helping people to lose weight has shown that when people lose weight, many of these problems, particularly the physical health problems, improve and can disappear.

Not having to take as many medicines can make a massive difference to a person's life. Prescriptions can be expensive and it can be frustrating if you have to take a lot of tablets every day. Losing weight can help you feel better and make your life easier.

Physical Health Problems

Heart Disease:

In an obese person, the heart has to pump much harder than it does in a healthy-weight person, and therefore obese people have a higher risk of heart attacks and strokes. When the heart struggles to cope in this way, the person can become tired, become short of breath, and can retain fluid, particularly in the legs.

Blood Clots:

The more obese you are, the more common blood clots become. Obese people tend to be less mobile and active than those who are a healthy weight. Although the most common place to get a blood clot is in the deep veins in the legs, sometimes these blood clots can travel to the lungs (known as a pulmonary embolism), which can be fatal. Blood clots in the legs form when the muscles in the legs do not pump the blood back to the heart and the blood sits still. The best way to prevent this is to walk around, which makes the muscles work, although wearing tight hospital or flight stockings can also help.

High Cholesterol:

Eating foods that are high in saturated fats can cause high blood cholesterol levels. High cholesterol increases the risk of heart attacks and strokes. It is important to reduce the amount of fat, particularly saturated fat, in your diet and to take medications, to help decrease this risk if your cholesterol is high.

Type 2 Diabetes:

Over 80 percent of people with obesity may develop Type 2 diabetes during their lifetime. This is also known as 'late onset' diabetes and the main cause of this is being overweight. Diabetes is a condition where your body cannot use the insulin produced in your pancreas gland to regulate the body's blood sugar. Having high blood sugar causes damage to your kidneys, nerves and your eyes. It is not uncommon for people with Type 2 diabetes to need amputations as the diabetes also causes damage to the blood vessels, which prevents blood flowing properly. Most people with Type 2 diabetes need to take daily medications and sometimes insulin injections. In many cases, when a person with Type 2 diabetes loses weight, their diabetes improves and they may no longer need to take insulin, or can reduce their medications. It is important not to do this unless you are told to do so by a doctor.

Sleep Apnoea:

If someone has sleep apnoea, it means that his or her breathing is interrupted during sleep, and in some cases, can even stop. Most people with sleep apnoea snore loudly, or their partner may notice them not breathing for a few seconds. This condition can make people feel very tired and sleepy during the day, and can cause severe headaches. If you are diagnosed with sleep apnoea, you may be given a mask attached to a machine (a CPAP machine) to wear at night. This is a tight fitting mask which forces air into your lungs, keeping your airways open. In most cases, once a person loses weight, their sleep apnoea improves or disappears.

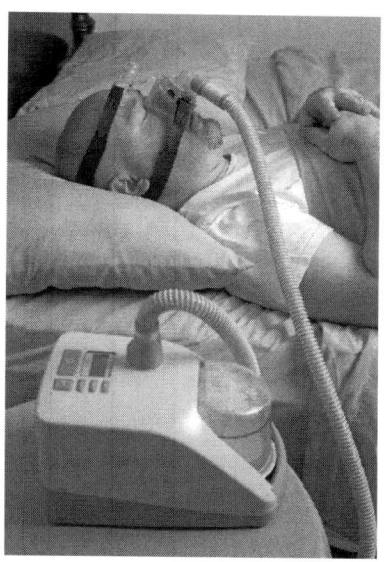

Arthritis and Back Pain:

The extra weight caused by being obese has to be carried by the back and the joints. This extra weight puts massive strain on your skeleton, and can cause arthritis, particularly of the hips and knees. This also puts pressure on the back, tightening the muscles, squeezing the disks in between the backbones and causing pain. Sometimes the pain in the back and joints can be so severe that people are unable to walk and need to take pain relief medications. It is often difficult for obese people to get knee or hip replacements, due to the risks these operations pose to someone who is obese. Although losing weight will not reverse arthritis, it will help reduce pain, and allow people to have replacement operations if necessary.

Infertility:

Obesity is also known to affect fertility. Many people, both men and women, with obesity find it very difficult to conceive. This is sometimes because the physical act of sex can become difficult when a person is very obese, but also the hormonal changes that occur in the body because of obesity may result in reduced fertility. In a significant number of cases, once a person loses weight, they find fertility significantly improves and women become pregnant much more easily.

Skin Problems:

People with obesity get chaffing of their legs, breasts, and arms and underneath their stomach. This can make this skin raw and very painful. They also sweat much more. Skin is often greasy, which leads to acne or painful spots on the back and breasts in particular. Skin infections become more common and can be difficult to treat. Again, the best way to reduce these problems is by losing weight.

Liver Disease:

Obese people often have a large fatty liver, which may eventually lead to liver disease. The liver is important in removing toxins and waste products from the body, so if the liver is diseased, these waste products build up and can cause severe illness. The liver also produces factors that help with blood clotting. People with liver disease often bleed very easily, which can be life threatening.

Cancer:

Obesity is known to increase the risks of certain types of cancer, particularly cancer of the oesophagus, breast, uterus, bowel, gallbladder, kidneys, pancreas, and thyroid gland.

Mental Health Problems

Obesity causes many problems with the way people view themselves. Many people become obese because they have had problems in their past, which may be depression, eating disorders or physical/sexual abuse. Some people may eat excessively to try to make themselves feel better. This is called "comfort eating" or "emotional eating". For some people, it is important that the appropriate psychological support is provided, such as seeing a counsellor, psychologist, or psychiatrist, as weight loss may not always help mental health problems.

Depression and Anxiety:

Depression is very common in obese people. Often, people become depressed or anxious because they are obese, they are unhappy with how they look, they feel bad about themselves, or because of things other people have said about them. People with obesity often feel discriminated against or stigmatised because of their weight. In these cases, helping people to lose weight can often improve their quality of life as well as their physical health problems. Sometimes simple depression treatments can make people feel better, but in other cases, the only way to cure their depression is by helping them to lose weight.

Eating Disorders:

Eating disorders are common in obese people. Many people with obesity suffer with bulimia (deliberately vomiting after eating). Binge eating is particularly common. This is when someone eats a significantly larger amount of food in one sitting than they normally would. Binge eating at night (night eating syndrome) is also common. If you suffer from an eating disorder, you should seek help from your doctor, a counsellor or psychologist.

Agoraphobia (fear of going outside):

Agoraphobia is common in obese people. When they go outside, they feel that people are staring at them and they are stigmatised. Most people who are overweight report times in their lives when they have felt discriminated against. Individuals can be extremely rude and mean about obese people, and can stare at or bully them. As a result, obese people can become scared of leaving their home. This leads to depression and anxiety.

It is always worth considering seeing a psychologist or doctor for any mental health problems, as there are many effective treatments today. However, there is certainly a link between obesity and mental health problems, many of which can be successfully treated with weight loss.

Should I Seek Help for My Weight?

Weight-loss surgery is becoming increasingly common. Weight-loss surgery can be an effective tool for people who have tried diets, exercise, and slimming tablets, but are still unable to lose significant amounts of weight and maintain the weight loss achieved.

This chapter has described many of the common health problems that are caused by obesity. If you are reading this book, it suggests that you are already thinking it is time to do something about your weight. You may already have some of the problems related to obesity, or you may simply be concerned that if you do not lose weight, you may develop some of these problems in the future.

Either way, reading this book is an important first step towards gaining control of your weight and health. Weight loss is not easy, and keeping it off is also very difficult. However, with the help of doctors, nurses, dietitians, friends, and family, weight does not need to control your life.

You can speak to your doctor about your local weight management programmes, or you can search for these yourself. A detailed and comprehensive package to help you lose weight as well as help to find a surgeon to discuss weight-loss surgery in detail can be found at **simply**bariatrics.com

Ultimately the decision of whether or not to have weight-loss surgery is up to you. Although many people who have struggled for years with their weight find surgery a good option, it is not right for everybody, and it is certainly not a magic cure. Support and advice are available at **simply**bariatrics.com to help whilst you make the long-term lifestyle changes that you will need to keep to have safe, successful long-term weight loss and maintenance.

Chapter 2
Diets and Consequences of Dieting

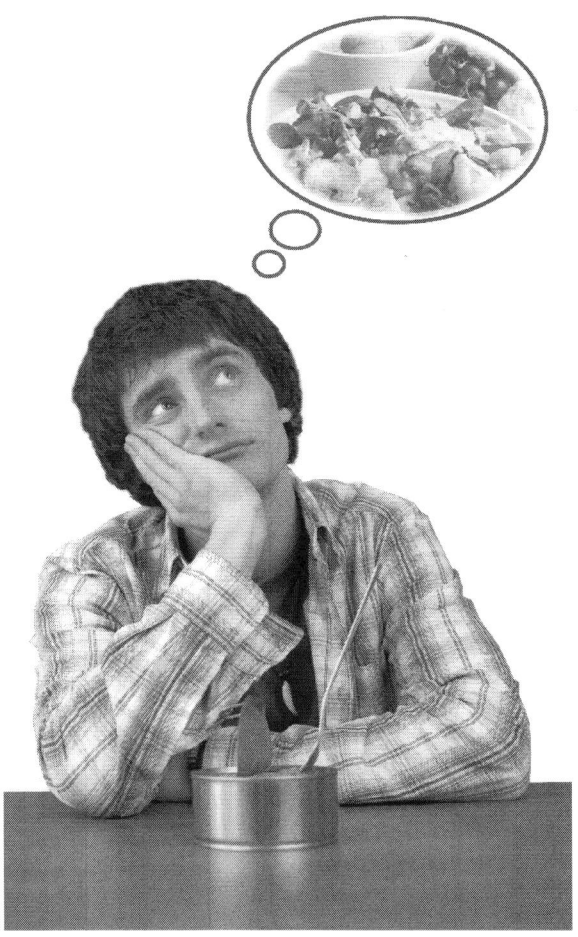

There are many commercial weight-loss diets and programmes that people have tried, on and off over many years. These diets have varying degrees of success, depending upon a person's motivation for weight loss and how easily the diet fits in with their usual lifestyle.

The Atkins diet is a low-carbohydrate diet, which was very popular a few years ago. However the British Dietetic Association, the American Heart Association and other professional health groups do not recommend it for the general public because of the long-term safety of the diet.

High-protein diets usually result in rapid weight loss due to the diuretic effect (fluid loss). It potentially limits the volume of food eaten, by reducing appetite and causing the dieter to feel fuller quicker, so high protein diets are likely to aid compliance.

Vitamin and mineral supplements are essential to ensure nutritional adequacy of some weight-loss diets. The high-protein and low-carbohydrate diets restrict fruit, vegetables, and wholegrain foods, which have been shown to be beneficial to health. More protein in the diet can lead to calcium loss, increasing the risk of developing osteoporosis. High-protein diets are not suitable for people with kidney disease or gout. It seems wise to seek a doctor's advice on the likely benefits and disadvantages of using a novel diet in order to lose weight.

It is not always the new diet that causes weight loss; it is usually the overall reduction in calories eaten that leads to the weight loss. In the longer term changes in lifestyle, eating habits, physical activity, and daily routine will contribute to long-term, weight-loss success. Just following a specific diet will not work in the long term.

Can Medically Unsupervised Diets Make You Obese?

Being on a strict diet can distort the mind and the body. This is because most of these diets involve giving up entire food types. Some call for eating nothing else except meat, meat products and salads. Such monotonous ways of eating can be unhealthy and can only work in the short term.

Diets that restrict calorie intake too much or cut out entire food groups such as carbohydrates can encourage the body to conserve fat. The body requires a minimum amount of nutrients each day. If we don't take enough nutrients from food, our bodies compensate by slowing down our metabolic rate to conserve energy. In other words, we stop burning fat.

Restricted eating can also prompt the body to break down muscle as a source of nutrients, and breaking down muscle causes the body to lose excess fluids. It is the combination of losing muscle and fluids that will show impressive results when getting on the scales.

The problem with losing muscle is that the ability to burn off any extra calories from food is reduced. This is because muscles are the part of our body that burns off more energy (calories). So, despite the promising initial weight loss, the end result may be the same amount of fat in the body and a greater tendency to weight gain in the long-term.

Other Weight Loss Strategies

There are many other strategies available to lose weight if dieting is a struggle. Different people find different things successful; some work for some people but may not work for everyone. Remember: the healthiest (and most successful long term) way to lose weight is a good diet combined with exercise.

Medications:

There have been a number of weight-loss medications, but none of these are 'magic weight-loss pills'. They work by preventing the absorption of the fat we eat. They work best when taken alongside a healthy balanced diet. Not all drugs are available in all countries; check with your doctor or local pharmacist for advice on which, if any, may be suitable for you.

> Orlistat (Alli)- Prevents absorption of fat, which is passed in the stool. Side effects include oily diarrhoea and leakage of oil from the bowels.
> Lorcaserin (Belviq)- Acts on receptors in the brain, making you feel full more quickly. Cannot be taken with

> certain anti-depressant medications. Causes tiredness, headache, constipation and cough.
>
> Phentermine-topiramate (Qsymia)- Makes you feel full and food less appetizing. Can lead to birth defects if taken during pregnancy. Other side effects include alterations in taste, dizziness, and tingling in hands and feet.

Other medications such as sibutramine have been removed from production due to serious, unwanted side effects.

Hypnotherapy:

Hypnotherapy can help some people lose weight by helping them to subconsciously overcome the desire to overeat. Using relaxation techniques, the hypnotherapist can help access the subconscious part of the mind and explore feelings about food, and what causes overeating. They can suggest new ways of thinking about food, which can help better control eating habits.

Hypnotherapy will NOT:

- cause someone to lose control
- put someone to sleep
- erase memories
- force someone to do something they don't want to do

- tell someone to do something they don't want to do

People will always be able to make their own choices; hypnotherapy can simply help with controlling the desire to over-eat and making someone think more about food choices or the way they eat.

Emotion Focused Therapy (EFT):

EFT involves psychotherapy with a trained counsellor. It usually consists of a course of sessions where the therapist helps explore and change any emotions that may cause overeating. They can then help develop strategies, which may help to avoid those negative emotions, or find new ways of coping with these emotions without involving food.

More information about these types of therapy can be found on **simply***bariatrics*.com or online in your local area.

Chapter 3
Am I Suitable for Weight-Loss (Bariatric) Surgery?

With the increasing prevalence of obesity, people are becoming more aware of weight-loss surgery as a means of losing significant amounts of weight and keeping their weight off in the longer term.

Losing weight improves a number of obesity related medical problems including diabetes, hypertension, asthma and other medical conditions. Weight-loss surgery, has been found to be the most effective means of weight loss and weight maintenance. So, how are suitable candidates for bariatric surgery identified?

Weight-loss surgery is indicated in people who have a body mass index (BMI) of over 40Kg/m2 or have a BMI equal or greater than 35Kg/m2 with medical conditions like type 2 diabetes, hypertension, obstructive sleep apnoea and others.

In addition:

1. Patients should have tried all other means of weight loss before considering weight-loss surgery, such as diets, exercise and weight loss drug therapy.

2. Patients should not have any life threatening illness, untreated psychiatric illness, or untreated eating disorders.

3. Patients should have been worked up by a specialist team comprising of a bariatric physician, dietitian, psychologist and bariatric surgeon who would assess suitability for surgery and the most suitable type of bariatric surgery.

4. Patients should have been assessed by an anaesthetist and deemed safe for surgery.

5. Patients should be prepared to change their life style and eating habits.

6. Patients should commit to regular follow up with a dietitian, surgeon, physician and psychologist.

7. It helps if patients have good support at home and attend a support group in the community.

Patients should be aware that bariatric surgery is not a magic cure. People can regain weight if they do not follow up at regular intervals and follow the advice provided. To learn more about the different bariatric surgical procedures and to understand what predicts a successful candidate, read all the relevant articles at the **simply***bariatrics*.com website.

Weight loss or bariatric surgery is recommended as a last option when all other non- surgical methods of weight loss have been tried for some time and failed.

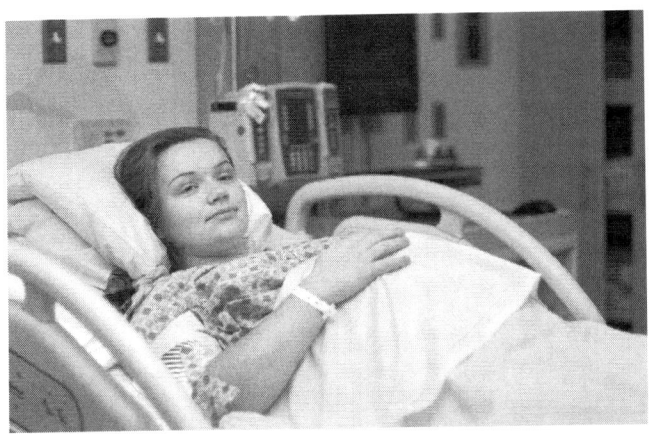

Guidelines for Weight-Loss Surgery

There are various sets of international guidelines that determine whether or not you are suitable for weight-loss surgery. In the UK, the National Institute of Health and Clinical Excellence (NICE) provides guidelines for new treatments based on clinical and cost effectiveness. Similar sets of guidelines exist in the US and Europe. According to NICE criteria, a patient will be recommended for bariatric surgery, if:

- their body mass index (BMI) is greater than or equal to 40 or 35-39 kg/m^2 with serious disease (e.g. type 2 diabetes or hypertension) that could be improved by weight loss.

- all appropriate non-surgical measures have been tried and failed to achieve or maintain adequate clinically beneficial weight loss for at least six months.

- they have been receiving or will receive intensive management in a specialist obesity service.

- they are generally fit for anaesthesia and surgery.

- they commit to long term follow-up.

Bariatric surgery is also recommended as a first line option (instead of lifestyle interventions or drug treatment) for adults with a BMI of more than 50 kg/m^2 in whom surgical intervention is considered appropriate.

Bariatric surgery is a cost effective treatment; however, there are still regional differences in the number of bariatric surgeries performed. This is due to local policies, expertise, funding availability, and the priorities of the commissioners and clinicians.

Development of guidelines alone does not help improve the availability of bariatric surgery to those in need. There should be appropriate funding and expertise. Long-term success of bariatric surgery depends on proper selection of patients and structured follow up. All bariatric centres should have a multidisciplinary team comprised of bariatric physicians, surgeons, dietitians, clinical psychologists, and physiotherapists, who select and support patients throughout their weight loss journey.

Government (State) Funded Bariatric Surgery

This will vary from country to country. Each country will have its own criteria for surgery. However, these are generally very similar.

In the UK, the National Health Service (NHS) has strict criteria as to who should be considered for bariatric surgery. This is based mainly upon evidence from the National Institute for Health and Clinical Excellence (NICE) obesity clinical guideline (CG)43.

The NHS will consider people for bariatric surgery if they have a BMI equal to or greater than 40kg/m^2 or a BMI of 35kg/m^2 or above with health problems associated with their weight. People must have tried and exhausted all other weight loss methods before being considered.

The medical problems that are generally considered to be obesity related include:

- High blood pressure
- Type 2 diabetes
- Obstructive sleep apnoea

- Significant arthritis or back/knee problems
- Depression

These have been described in more detail in Chapter 1.

Many patients with obesity suffer from depression and/or anxiety, or have problems in their past that mean they may need a little more support adjusting to surgery. Some people may need to see a psychologist before they have surgery. This is to make sure that they get the support required through their weight-loss surgery journey and have safe, successful long-term weight loss.

Most areas will require people to have attended a local community weight-management programme before being referred for bariatric surgery. These programmes have doctors, dietitians, psychologists, nurses and exercise therapists to assess, advise and monitor a person's progress. These weight-management programmes can vary in length and can last for up to two years. It is usually the staff in these programmes or a GP that will decide if a person is suitable for consideration for bariatric surgery.

Some areas have in the past had higher BMI referral criteria for bariatric surgery on the NHS, such as a BMI of 45kg/m^2 and above with an obesity related medical problem or BMI 50kg/m^2 and above. However, recent commissioning changes should have largely ironed out these differences. A General Practitioner (GP) or community weight management programme will have information on what the local bariatric surgery NHS referral criteria and referral processes are.

Bariatric Surgery in Private Hospitals (Self-Funded)

In the UK private health care sector, people who pay for bariatric surgery themselves can be considered for bariatric surgery if they have a BMI equal to or greater than 40kg/m^2 or 35kg/m^2 and above with health problems associated with their weight, as per NICE CG43 guidance.

In the US and some European countries it is now deemed acceptable to offer surgery to people with a BMI between 30 and 35kg/m^2 and many UK surgeons will also consider performing bariatric surgery on people with a BMI in this range, depending upon the individual's circumstances and health.

People who wish to self-fund their bariatric surgery will be assessed by a surgeon and a dietitian or nurse. They should still have demonstrated that they have tried other weight-loss methods.

People who self-fund their surgery do not have to have attended a community weight-management programme and therefore this can significantly reduce the length of time between being assessed by a surgeon and a dietitian or nurse and having bariatric surgery.

People who are self-funding their bariatric surgery generally do not have to wait for long before having their surgery. Usually, they can also decide an operation date that is convenient to them.

There are a number of bariatric surgery packages available from many different companies. It is important to consider and choose the right company, surgeon, and aftercare package that meets your needs. See "How to Choose a Surgeon/ Hospital" or see the **simply***bariatrics*.com website for more information.

When is Weight-Loss Surgery Not Recommended?

Criteria for bariatric surgery vary between different hospitals and countries. Criteria are also different between public and private hospitals. The standard criteria followed by most centres include a body mass index (BMI) of 40kg/m2 or above or a BMI of 35 to 40kg/m2 with weight-related medical problems. The aim of performing weight-loss surgery is to improve or prevent medical problems. In the UK and other countries bariatric surgery is now considered first line treatment if the BMI is more than 50kg/m2.

Bariatric surgery is not recommended if you are found unsuitable for general anaesthesia or you cannot give consent for the operation.

There are several other conditions where bariatric surgery is not recommended:

1. If the patient has life-threatening illness, including terminal cancers, severe renal (kidney) failure, liver failure, and heart failure.
2. If the patient has untreated eating disorders.
3. If the patient has untreated or severe psychiatric illness.

In addition, the success of weight-loss surgery in people with obesity related to genetic causes is debatable. For example, bariatric surgery for people with Prader-Willi syndrome and MC4R deficiency has not been successful in the long term.

Chapter 4
Different Types of Weight-Loss Surgery

There are a number of different types of weight loss operations, all of which have advantages and disadvantages. It is important to research each type of surgery and talk to a surgeon and a dietitian before making a decision about which one to go for.

Broadly speaking, weight loss procedures can be split into a number of categories:

- **Reversible:** Endobarrier, gastric balloon, gastric band
- **Irreversible:** gastric bypass, sleeve gastrectomy, biliopancreatic diversion/duodenal switch
- **Restrictive:** (prevents people from eating large volumes of food)- gastric balloon, gastric band, sleeve gastrectomy
- **Malabsorptive:** Endobarrier
- **Restrictive *and* malabsorptive:** gastric bypass, biliopancreatic diversion/duodenal switch
- **Need a general anaesthetic:** Endobarrier, gastric band, gastric bypass, sleeve gastrectomy, biliopancreatic diversion/duodenal switch
- **Done under local anaesthesia/sedation-** gastric balloon, Endobarrier

A surgeon performing a bariatric operation.

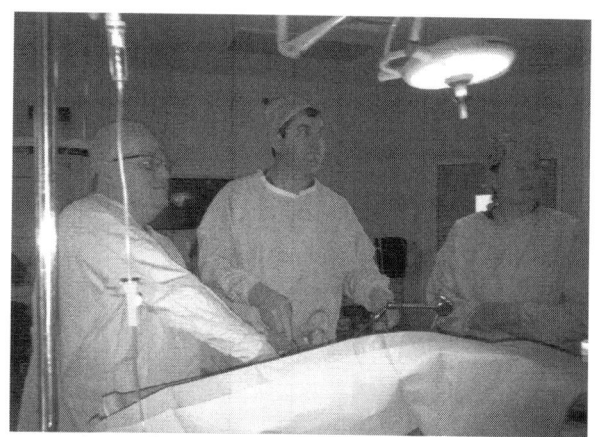

There are a number of weight-loss procedures available. The most common procedures are gastric band, sleeve gastrectomy, and gastric bypass. The biliopancreatic diversion and duodenal switch are not performed routinely because of the high number of complications. There are newer procedures such as the Endobarrier (also known as the endo sleeve), gastric plication and POSE, but there are no long-term results/data from these procedures and they are not routinely performed.

This chapter will describe each of the common operations in detail, and will help you decide which is the right procedure for you.

Intra-gastric Balloon

The intra-gastric balloon is a removable device that works by reducing the amount you can eat. The gastric balloon, which is like a rubber ball filled with fluid, sits in the body of the stomach, making you feel full more quickly and therefore stops you from eating a large meal. The reduction in calories, will lead to more weight loss.

Once the balloon is placed, it stays in for up to six months, before it is removed. The main advantage of the gastric balloon is that neither insertion nor removal requires an anaesthetic. The procedure is performed by a doctor qualified in endoscopy (this does not have to be a surgeon), and can be done with or without sedation. It takes around 30 minutes and can be performed as an out-patient procedure. This means you can go home usually about an hour after it has been placed or removed, and do not have to stay in hospital.

When you arrive for your appointment, the doctor will spray your throat with some local anaesthetic, and possibly give you some sedation. This will not put you to sleep, but will make you feel more relaxed and less anxious. The doctor will look down into your stomach with a camera (perform an endoscopy) and then remove it. The balloon is then fed down into your stomach through your mouth in the same way. In most cases, the doctor will then put the camera back down into the stomach so that they can check that the balloon is sitting in the right place before it is inflated.

The balloon is attached to a syringe that allows the doctor to inflate it with fluid. The fluid usually contains a blue dye, which, if the fluid were to leak, would turn your urine blue. This dye does not cause you any harm, but lets the doctor know the balloon has burst. Once the balloon is inflated, the camera and the syringe tubing are removed and you are taken through to recovery.

The gastric balloon does not make you lose as much weight as most other procedures, and is often used to help very obese people lose a bit of weight before they have another operation (i.e. the gastric bypass). It could be useful however if you only want to lose a small amount of weight.

Gastric Band

The gastric band works by restricting the amount you can eat. The gastric band is fitted around the stomach, just below the top of it. The gastric band is filled with fluid, and the part of the stomach above the band (the 'pouch') is where food sits whilst it is digested. This means that you feel full very quickly, and anything you eat has to be digested and pass out of the pouch, through the gastric band, before you can eat anything else.

The gastric band is fitted during a keyhole (laparoscopic) operation. There are usually about four or five small wounds for the surgeon to place the instruments they need into the abdomen. The surgeon makes a tunnel behind the stomach, and fits the gastric band around it. Above the gastric band, the stomach forms a 'pouch' which is around the size of an egg-cup, and once this pouch is full, you will feel like you cannot eat any more until the food has passed through the gastric band. Once the surgeon has placed the gastric band in the correct position, it is fastened, and stitched in place to try and stop it from moving or 'slipping'.

Attached to the gastric band is some tubing that allows fluid to be injected into the gastric band, adjusting how tight it is, allowing more or less food to pass through. The surgeon will pull this tubing out of one of the small key holes they have made in the abdomen, usually just below the ribs on the left side. They then close the rest of the wounds in the abdomen with stitches, staples or glue. The gastric band port is placed underneath the skin and fastened to the band tubing, then stitched to the abdominal wall. The skin on top of it is closed in the same way as the other wounds. People usually only need to stay in hospital overnight after having a gastric band fitted, and some people may even go home on the same day if they are well enough.

The tightness of the gastric band can be adjusted via the port that is placed under the skin on the abdominal wall. Some people prefer having the band very tight, which makes them eat less textured food, but it may be higher in soft, easier-to-tolerate calories. If the gastric band is a little looser, people find that they can make better dietary choices, which are lower in calories. You should communicate with the bariatric team about this when you go to get the gastric band filled with fluid. The less you eat, the more weight you will lose, but it is important to eat a healthy diet to maintain your health.

The gastric band can be taken out if you experience any problems. Removing the band requires another operation, but some people prefer to have the band because it can be reversed in the future.

The other big advantage of the gastric band is that because none of the stomach is removed or stapled, it is still able to produce all of the hormones and enzymes that your body needs to digest your food and keep the body healthy. You may still need to take vitamin and mineral supplements, but you will not have the side effects, such as diarrhoea and dumping syndrome, associated with other weight loss operations.

Sleeve Gastrectomy

The gastric sleeve, or sleeve gastrectomy, works by reducing the volume of food that you can eat at any one time and is very successful in aiding weight loss.

The sleeve is usually performed by keyhole (laparoscopic) surgery. There are usually about four or five small wounds made, through which the surgeon places the instruments they need into the abdomen. The surgeon inserts a tube down your throat into your stomach, and then uses his instruments to push this tube so it sits along the inner (or 'lesser') curve of your stomach. A stapling device is then used to staple along this tube, disconnecting most of the stomach and leaving a thin sleeve of stomach, which is still connected to your oesophagus and bowel at either end. The rest of the stomach is then removed and the wounds closed with stitches, staples, or glue. Sometimes the surgeon will use a buttressing material or special glue on your stomach, which helps to stop the stapled area from bleeding or leaking.

The thin tube of stomach, or "sleeve", is where food sits whilst it is digested. As the sleeve is so narrow, you feel full after a very small amount of food. The sleeve is called a 'restrictive' operation (meaning you can't eat as much because you feel full quickly). The stomach also produces many of the digestive enzymes you need to digest and absorb food. As most of the stomach is removed, the production of these enzymes is reduced, and you therefore may not be able to absorb as much food as before the surgery.

There are very few long-term complications with the sleeve gastrectomy, so once you have recovered from surgery, it is rare for you to experience significant problems. The sleeve is a permanent operation, so you do not have to attend the hospital for adjustments like you do with the gastric band. You need to stay in the hospital for about two to three days after the operation. You will be seen by a dietitian, who will go through what you can and cannot eat after surgery.

Gastric Bypass

The gastric bypass is a very successful weight-loss operation. Although the other operations are also very effective, people tend to lose more weight after the gastric bypass. This is very useful in diabetic patients, and has the best chance of getting rid of your diabetes. Some people also find that they no longer like sweet foods after gastric bypass, which can be useful if you have a sweet tooth!

The gastric bypass is both a 'restrictive' and a 'malabsorptive' procedure, which works by reducing the volume of food that you can eat at any one time, and also by stopping you from absorbing some of the nutrition that you eat. It is usually performed by laparoscopic (keyhole) surgery, unless you have any other abdominal problems, or have had a large abdominal operation in the past. During surgery, the surgeon makes five or six small wounds for the instruments. The majority of your stomach is disconnected from the oesophagus (food pipe), leaving a small eggcup sized or golf ball pouch. This pouch is where food initially sits before moving on into the bowel. As the pouch is so small, you feel full after a very small amount of food. Some of the small bowel is then disconnected, usually one to two metres downstream from the stomach. Where the small bowel has been disconnected, the surgeon brings the bottom part of the small bowel (which is still connected to the large bowel) up and connects it to the pouch of stomach at the bottom of the oesophagus.

This means that the rest of the stomach, and the top part of small bowel are initially not connected to anything. The surgeon measures down from the join between the stomach pouch and small bowel, and reconnects the loose bit of stomach and small bowel to the rest of the small bowel. When you eat, the food passes down the oesophagus, through the small pouch of stomach, and down the small bowel. Part way down the small bowel, the food is joined by all of the digestive juices from the stomach, liver, and pancreas, and after this, digestion is normal. This operation means that only part of your small bowel can absorb food.

Although the gastric bypass is a complicated operation, there are only a small number of long-term complications that occur, and therefore it is a very good long-term operation.

Biliopancreatic Diversion (BPD)

This procedure is essentially a variant of the roux-en-y gastric bypass. However the gastric pouch is much larger than in the standard bypass (approximately one third of the stomach). The remaining two thirds of the stomach is usually removed. The small bowel is then divided much lower down than with a bypass. The BPD is therefore more malabsorptive and less restrictive than the standard bypass. This means that you can eat more but may get loose bowel motions.

Duodenal Switch (DS)

This is a variant of the BPD. The operation begins with a sleeve gastrectomy in which two-thirds to three-quarters of the stomach are removed. The duodenum (first part of the small bowel) is then divided. The small bowel is also divided much lower down, close to the caecum (where the small bowel joins the large bowel). The small bowel beyond the divide is joined on to the duodenum, which is still connected to the stomach. The rest of the small bowel is plumbed in lower down. As with a BPD, this procedure is more malabsorptive and less restrictive than the bypass.

Many surgical procedures can help you lose weight. However, none of these procedures does all of the work for you. It is very important that you change your eating habits and lifestyle if you are considering weight-loss surgery, or the procedure will not work effectively and you will regain weight in the long-term.

The **simply**bariatrics.com website contains more information, and videos of each of these operations which you should watch. It is also worth reading about the experiences of patients who have had surgery in the past, as these are the best people to explain what to expect. If you have any further questions, speak to your doctor, surgeon, or bariatric team.

Comparison of Weight-loss Surgery Operations

Making the decision to have surgery is a huge step. Once committed to surgery, there are three main types of weight-loss surgery to consider. To get a copy of a table comparing different weight loss surgeries please email us at hello@simplybariatrics.com

Chapter 5
How to Arrange Bariatric Surgery

Before considering bariatric surgery, it is a good idea to undertake some research and look at some books, online forums, and websites. Websites often have links to clinics and hospitals, which recommend surgeons and bariatric surgery services.

In most cases, whether seeking surgery through a healthcare system such as the NHS, or self-funding the operation; it is a good idea to discuss this with your General Practitioner or family doctor. They often know of good surgeons and services and can recommend someone with an excellent track record. They often know the local hospitals, and can help make the decision to go for surgery. In most cases, your doctor will have to write a referral letter to the hospital or consultant before you can see the bariatric team.

The referral pathway will vary from country to country. In some countries surgeons are directly accessible. In others, a referral is needed from your family doctor. In the UK, all NHS patients now have to be referred for surgery via a local community weight-management programme. Local weight management programmes can be found online and patients can usually refer themselves.

In the local community weight-management programmes, they will cover dietary and lifestyle changes, exercise, and other ways to improve your health. In most cases you will see a dietitian. You can often get discounts to gyms, or take part in exercise programmes. If you suffer from depression or any other mental health problem, see a counsellor or psychologist. This can be essential in helping the patient to lose as much weight as possible.

As long as the patient engages with the community weight management programme, show that they are committed to losing weight, and fulfil the NICE CG43 or local BMI criteria they will then usually be referred to a bariatric surgery service. The next step is an appointment to see the surgeon and/or dietitian, nurse and psychologist at the hospital. Some hospitals ask that you attend an education seminar at the hospital before you see the surgeon; here they will discuss bariatric surgery in more detail and make sure that you wish to go ahead.

How to Choose a Surgeon

It is important to make sure your surgeon has the appropriate qualifications. In the UK, the surgeon should be registered with the General Medical Council (GMC- you can check this on their website) and be a Fellow of one of the Royal Colleges of Surgeons

(FRCS) and be a member of the British Obesity and Metabolic Surgery Society (BOMSS).

They will need to hold a CCT (Certificate of Completion of Training) or CCST (Certificate of Completion of Specialist Training). They should have a specialist interest in bariatric surgery, meaning they perform at least 50 bariatric surgery operations per year and work in a centre that performs at least 125 operations per year.

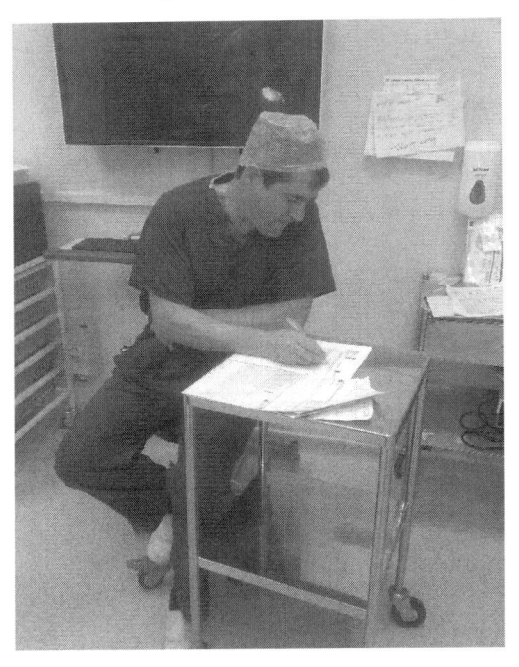

Surgeon writing post-operative notes

In the US, ensure your surgeon is board certified and that he or she is a member of the American Society for Metabolic and Bariatric Surgery (ASMBS). They should be working in a hospital that performs at least 125 bariatric surgery operations per year. In other European countries, the surgeon must be appropriately qualified and registered and fulfil the same number criteria as above.

How to Choose a Surgeon in a Private Setting

If you are considering having bariatric surgery privately you should be able to book an appointment directly to see the surgeon and dietitian/nurse for an assessment and advice at a private hospital. Some surgeons may prefer to have a referral letter from a doctor prior to seeing them. You should check with the hospital or private company when you are booking your consultation appointment. Once the surgeon has performed an assessment and discussed your bariatric surgery options they will then inform your GP that you are considering or are planning to have bariatric surgery.

How to Choose the Right Hospital

A team of dedicated health care professionals and a well-equipped hospital are important for uncomplicated and successful weight-loss surgery.

In addition to a bariatric surgeon, the team should include an experienced anaesthetist who specifically has plenty of experience in anaesthesia for obese people. Other members of the team should include a specialist bariatric dietitian, a specialist bariatric nurse, a clinical psychologist with experience in obesity and weight-loss surgery and, in many cases, a bariatric physician.

A specialist unit should have trained staff who understand the problems and needs of individuals with weight problems. All staff should be trained in the moving and handling of obese people. You should be supported from the very first consultation. Look out to see if they have appropriate furniture including bariatric chairs, bariatric beds, hoists to help move you, walk-in showers, appropriate toilets, etc.

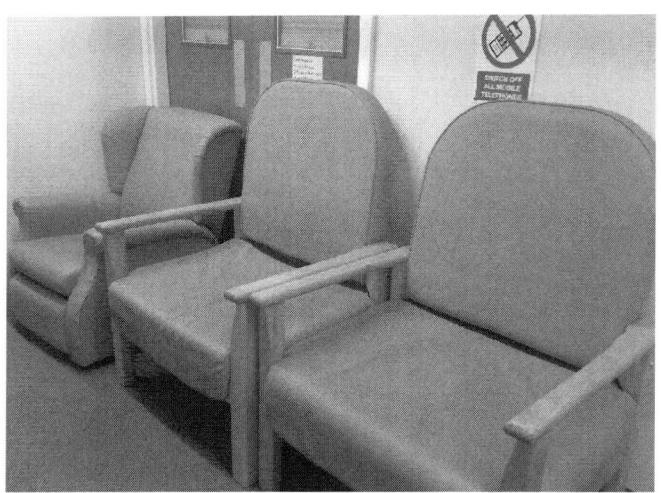

Bariatric chairs

A bariatric centre should be undertaking at least 125 bariatric procedures a year with each surgeon performing at least 50 bariatric surgeries in a year.

Find out from the hospital if they have:

1. A 24-hour emergency helpline if there is no accident and emergency department in the hospital.
2. A named person to talk to if there is a problem.
3. Details of the follow-up schedule after discharge from hospital.
4. Details of the service offered within the package, in the case of a private hospital.
5. A specialist bariatric team.
6. A patient support group, which runs at frequent intervals.
7. Bariatric equipment (chairs, beds, gowns, hoist, large blood pressure cuffs).
8. A comprehensive after care/support programme to ensure you have safe, successful, long-term weight loss.

It is also important to ensure the hospital you choose is, where possible, not very far away from where you live. You may want to visit this hospital for regular follow up or your family members would like to visit you whilst you are admitted.

You can check with your local hospital, either on-line or by calling, what their complication and death rates are. In the UK, you can check www.drfosterhealth.co.uk.

Do not be afraid to ask the surgeon about their complications, success and death rates. They should be honest and, if they refuse to answer, consider seeking an alternative surgeon.

Cost of Having Weight-Loss Surgery

Patients having state-funded surgery will not be expected to pay for either the operation or aftercare. You will have to buy your own equipment to use at home such as a food blender and nutritional supplements, but the hospital stay and follow-up care will be fully funded.

Prices in the private sector depend upon which bariatric operation you have, the aftercare package, and which company/surgeon you have chosen to perform the surgery.

It is very important to find out exactly what costs are involved in the entire weight-loss surgery process. This includes your hospital stay, how much after care will be needed, and other aspects such as the number of band adjustments included in the aftercare package. After care is probably the most important aspect of weight-loss surgery to ensure safe, successful, long-term weight loss. Therefore you should opt for the package that gives you the support you feel that you will require after surgery.

Consider how aftercare will be accessed, how often it occurs and whom it is with, such as the surgeon, dietitian or nurse. Check to see if there are accessible clinic appointments, send emails to the bariatric team with queries, and have telephone contact. Check to ensure that the aftercare is accessible, particularly if the hospital/service is not close to home. Whilst this may not be the cheapest option, it may be the best option in the long-term to ensure the expected weight loss and health benefits.

Health Tourism for Weight-Loss Surgery

People go to a foreign country to have weight-loss surgery for a number of the following reasons:

1. Lower cost of surgery in another country.
2. Surgery to be performed by an experienced surgeon based in another country.
3. Well-reputed hospital in a foreign country.
4. Patients do not meet criteria for surgery in home country.
5. Patients want to combine surgery with a holiday.

Those of you who have tried all measures to lose weight and have not been successful may start contemplating bariatric surgery. It is important to understand that it is not just the surgery which is important for long-term success. You should be supported before and long after you have had surgery by your bariatric team, family, and friends

However, health tourism is very popular, specifically to meet the needs of people who want to get treated away from home. There are many surgeons and good hospitals in other countries, where you may wish to get operated upon. Health care systems are varied and hence do not expect the same level of service and care that you will be provided in the UK. Do not get carried away by attractive advertisements and offers.

Before you decide to go abroad and have surgery, it is essential to gather as much information as possible.

Check List for Having Bariatric Surgery Abroad:

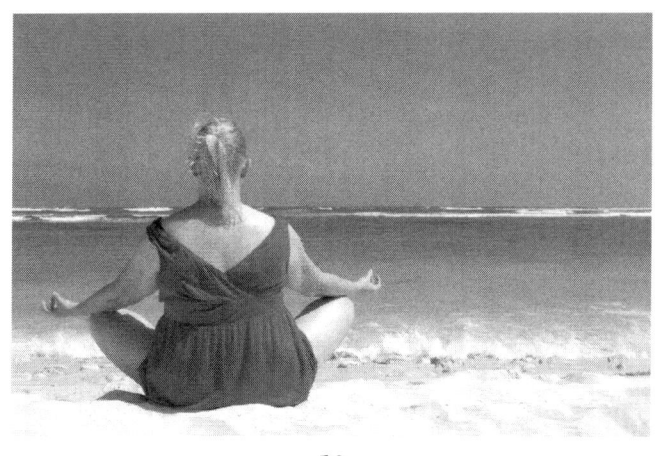

1. Is the hospital well equipped for bariatric surgery?
2. How many weight-loss surgeries are performed in a year?
3. What is the complication rate in the hospital?
4. How many bariatric surgeries has the surgeon performed?
5. Has anyone you know been to that hospital for surgery?
6. What is the follow up plan?
7. Who would look after you when you return?
8. Who will you contact when there is an emergency?
9. Is there accountability and a complaints system in that hospital?
10. Is a local surgeon available to follow-up with upon return?

Having bariatric surgery in a foreign country is a major decision and should not be taken lightly. Read related articles to learn more about follow-up care after bariatric surgery and how you could have bariatric surgery in the UK.

Chapter 6
Preparation for Bariatric Surgery

Making preparations before having a weight-loss surgery procedure is important to ensure expectations are clear before, during and after your procedure. Being prepared before surgery is the key to how successful weight loss will be in the long term. This chapter will help consider what preparation is needed before having bariatric surgery.

Discuss Bariatric Surgery Plans with Family & Friends

Some people want to tell the whole world of their plans for bariatric surgery, whilst others want to keep it to themselves. The decision of who to tell and who not to tell is personal, take time to consider who among family and friends needs to know and who doesn't.

It is important to consider discussing your plans for bariatric surgery with family and friends. Think about who you will inform and when. Decide who may be the most supportive of bariatric surgery and what they will need to know.

Sometimes it may be difficult to know how family and friends may react to the news. Be prepared for both positive and negative comments which you may receive, and lots of questions.

If time off from work is needed for the surgery and recovery, you should inform your manager or employer of your plans. Some people choose to take annual leave to avoid informing colleagues at work about having bariatric surgery.

Remember, not everyone may be supportive and some may be discouraging about having bariatric surgery or even try to sabotage weight loss efforts after surgery. Previous bariatric surgery patients report that some family and friends have been influenced by scare stories that they have read in magazines and newspapers or seen on the television. Most find that these people know little about the real facts about bariatric surgery and the positive health and quality of life outcomes that they experience.

Informing family and friends and discussing weight-loss surgery plans with them allows them to provide positive support during the weight loss journey.

Pre-Surgery Dietary and Lifestyle Changes

Once plans are in place for bariatric surgery, it is important not to put weight on by eating 'last suppers' and consuming foods that you think you may not ever be able to eat again. You need to show some commitment and motivation to make life-long lifestyle changes in preparation for bariatric surgery.

Before your operation, if you gain weight, do not lose weight or do not meet your weight loss target as advised by your bariatric centre, the surgeon may delay or cancel your operation. Most bariatric centres will require you to show that you have made attempts to lose weight. This may be from following weight-management programmes local to you or from attending or subscribing on the Internet to commercial slimming clubs.

It is important to start making dietary and lifestyle changes before having bariatric surgery. People who make changes and lose weight before surgery are more likely to have successful, long-term weight loss. Losing weight before surgery will not only reduce your anaesthetic risk but also make it easier to come to terms with the dietary and lifestyle changes that are required after surgery.

If you make some or all of these changes before surgery it will be easier to recover and develop lifelong, positive eating habits and eating patterns.

Dietary and lifestyle changes to consider making before surgery are:

- Plan and prepare meals ahead.
- Use a tea plate or smaller plate to serve your meals on.
- Avoid taking food and fluid together; leave 30 minutes before and after food.

- Establish a regular meal pattern, aiming for three meals per day.
- Include breakfast.
- Avoid eating late at night.
- Reduce or avoid snacking.
- Eat slowly and chew your food well.
- Avoid fizzy drinks and use reduced sugar and no added sugar drinks instead.
- Reduce or avoid drinking alcohol.
- Use artificial sweeteners rather than sugar.
- Increase your activity levels.
- Take a daily vitamin and mineral supplement if advised by your bariatric centre.

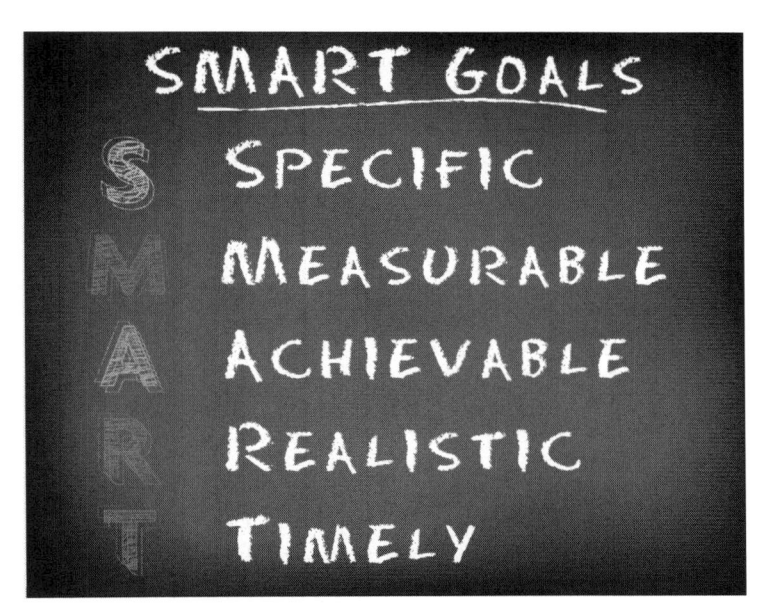

Setting SMART goals

Investigations Before Weight-Loss Surgery

Before you have surgery, your surgeon and anaesthetist may want you to have a number of investigations, to make sure that you are healthy and to make sure there are no problems on the day of surgery.

Blood Tests:

Your physician will carry out a thorough physical examination and order investigations to:

1. Ascertain that you do not have any serious medical or hormonal problems that may have resulted in weight gain.
2. Ensure you are safe to have anaesthesia and recovery from surgery is uneventful.

A number of blood tests may be requested, depending on the suspicion of endocrine (hormonal) problems including:

- Full Blood Count (FBC)
- Urea & Electrolytes (U&E)
- Liver Function Test (LFT)
- Thyroid Function Test (TFT)

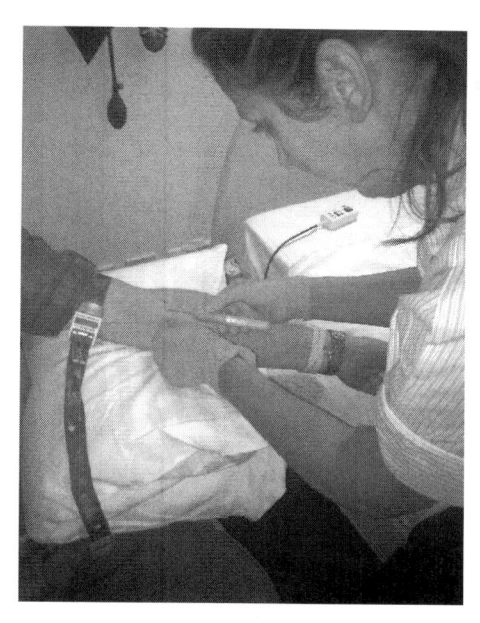

Pre-operative blood test

There are a number of blood tests that are taken before any operation. These are done to check how well your liver and kidneys are functioning, as surgery can occasionally put strain on them. They also check for anaemia (lack of red blood cells). Red blood cells carry oxygen around the body, and this keeps your cells and organs working properly. If red blood cell count is low, iron may be given (this helps the body produce more healthy cells) to take before your operation.

If there is a suspicion of other hormonal conditions, further tests will be ordered. For example, if your physician suspects Cushing's syndrome (a hormonal condition, where your body produces more than normal steroids), you will be asked to have series of urine and blood tests.

It is important before any weight-loss surgery operation to check that you are not already deficient in any vitamins or minerals. Some of the weight loss operations mean that after surgery, your body does not absorb nutrients (vitamins and minerals) as easily as before surgery, so it is important to make sure your levels are normal ***before*** the operation. If you are lacking in any of these important vitamins or minerals, you may be given nutritional supplements before surgery.

Gastroscopy:

Although not all surgeons require you to have one of these tests, you may be sent for a gastroscopy before your surgery. A gastroscopy involves putting a camera down your mouth and inspecting the inside of your oesophagus (food pipe), stomach and duodenum (first part of your small bowel). This is to make sure that you do not have a hiatus hernia or bacteria called H. Pylori living in your stomach.

A hiatus hernia is when the opening in your diaphragm (the sheet of muscle between your chest and abdomen) gets a little bigger than normal and part of the stomach can move up into your chest. This usually needs to be repaired before having weight-loss surgery.

H. Pylori is a type of bacteria that lives in the stomach. It is known to be associated with gastro-oesophageal reflux (heartburn) and has occasionally been known to cause stomach cancer in a very small number of patients. After bariatric surgery, it is thought that H. Pylori can increase the chances of getting a narrowing (known as a stricture) in the joins or staple lines in your stomach or bowel. If you are found to have H. Pylori, you will be given antibiotics to remove it before surgery. There are other tests that can be done to look for H. Pylori, but a gastroscopy is the most reliable.

Sleep Studies:

Many people with obesity suffer with sleep apnoea, a condition that causes interruption of breathing during sleep. Many people do not know they have sleep apnoea, but it is important to diagnose because you will be asleep during your surgery. You may be given a questionnaire to assess your risk of sleep apnoea, and some patients may be asked to go for sleep studies before surgery.

If you are diagnosed with sleep apnoea, you may be given a machine (called a CPAP machine), which is connected to a mask that you wear at night. This machine pushes air into your lungs, keeping the small airways at the bottom of your lungs open, making sure you can breathe easily.

Heart and Blood Pressure Readings:

It is important to make sure that your heart is working properly before you have a weight loss operation. You will have your heart rate checked and blood pressure readings taken. If necessary, medication may be given to make sure these are as normal as possible.

Other Tests:

You will probably be asked for a urine sample to make sure you have no infection before surgery, and to make sure that you have no undiagnosed diabetes. You will also have to have MRSA swabs before coming into the hospital for your operation. MRSA is a type of bacteria that lives on the skin of three in ten people. It usually doesn't cause any problems, but if it gets into a wound, it can cause an infection. If you are found to have MRSA, you will be given treatment before your operation.

All of the above tests are routine: do not worry about these tests, as most people having surgery need to have these done!

Dietary Preparation before Weight-loss surgery

Dietary preparation before weight-loss surgery, particularly for the liquid and pureed stage of the diet, is the key to ensuring that appropriate dietary advice and menu plans are followed. It will also ensure familiarity with the expected diet in the first few weeks after surgery.

This is particularly important in the first few weeks during recovery after surgery when you may not feel like preparing and cooking food.

You will need to follow a liquid and/or pureed diet for up to the first three to six weeks after your operation, depending upon the advice of your dietitian and bariatric centre. If you or someone else prepares this stage of the diet before your operation, it may be easier to understand and follow the appropriate diet, which will reduce the risk of having problems with vomiting and pain after eating.

A blender will be needed to puree food; this will ensure that there are no lumps or bits that are likely to become stuck and cause vomiting in the early stages after your operation. When the food has been pureed it can be placed in ice cube containers and frozen, ready for reheating after your operation.

Many people also use meal replacement drinks, smooth nutritious soups and smoothies whilst on the liquid and pureed stage of this diet. Meal replacement drinks provide suitable nutrition and can be more palatable than two to three tablespoons of pureed food for a meal. They are both good sources of nutrition and fluid. Some people feel more comfortable using these drinks in the early stages after surgery, as they are less likely to cause vomiting and pain.

Pre-Operative Liver Shrinkage Diet

Most bariatric surgery centres advise a preoperative 'liver shrinkage' diet running up to the operation date. There are a number of different preoperative 'liver shrinkage' diets that are advised by bariatric centres. The aim of these diets is to shrink the glycogen (carbohydrate) stores in your liver. The diet will also lead to weight loss.

Most people who meet the criteria for bariatric surgery will have a large, fatty liver. By following the advised pre-operative diet, the liver will reduce in size. The liver lies over the top of the stomach, so by reducing the size of the liver the surgeon is able to see the stomach more readily in order to perform the surgery laparoscopically (keyhole), which can also reduce the length of time of the operation.

The liver shrinkage diets include using meal replacement drinks, milk and yoghurt diet, a low-calorie diet, a meal-replacement diet or low-carbohydrate diet. The length of time you are advised to follow the diet also varies, from seven days to a few months. Sometimes the length of time you are advised to follow the diet may depend upon your BMI and/or general health.

Each bariatric service and surgeon will choose their preferred option, which they feel gives the best results in achieving liver shrinkage. It is important to stick to the diet that the surgeon and dietitian have chosen; ***do not*** choose any other diet or combine them.

If your liver remains large and fatty because you have not followed the diet, the surgeon may not be able to perform the operation. The surgeon may have intended to undertake the procedure laparoscopically (keyhole) but may decide that, due to your large liver size and the anaesthetic risk, an open procedure is more appropriate or not to perform the surgery at all. You could also have a different procedure to what was originally planned, such as a sleeve gastrectomy instead of a gastric bypass.

It is important to plan the liver shrinkage pre-operative diet ahead of the start date. This will allow time to make sure you and those around you know what the diet consists of and how to follow the diet. It will also give you the chance to check with the bariatric centre should you be unsure about anything. This may include ensuring that you purchase the appropriate yoghurts or meal replacement drinks and if any changes in your usual medication are required whilst following the diet.

You will also need to consider how you will manage this pre-operative diet during this time. There are several issues to consider:

- Will you be at work whilst on the diet?
- Do you prepare and cook meals for the family such as children and others?
- How you will spread your diet throughout the day? This may depend upon your usual routine such as work, shopping, meeting friends, childcare.
- Are there any meals out, parties, holidays, or celebrations planned during the pre-operative diet period?
- How will mealtimes and socialising with others be managed?
- How will medication be managed whilst following the diet?
- Consideration of how you will respond if someone questions why you are not eating with family, eating smaller portions, or drinking a meal replacement are important, particularly if you don't want people to know that you are having bariatric surgery.

Vitamin and Mineral Supplementation

Most bariatric centres recommend vitamin and mineral supplements after bariatric surgery. Some centres also advise you to take nutritional supplements before bariatric surgery and whilst on the pre-operative liver-shrinkage diet. The dietitian and bariatric centre should be able to advise you on suitable nutritional supplements to take and the dose required.

It is important to purchase the vitamin and mineral supplements that are recommended to you before you have the operation. You are likely to start taking the nutritional supplements within the first day or two after surgery, so you will need to take them into hospital with you.

Some bariatric centres advise chewable or dissolvable vitamin and mineral supplements during the liquid/pureed phase of the post-operative diet. Vitamin and mineral supplements can be large in size and therefore can be difficult to swallow in the first few weeks after surgery.

Medication

If you take any medication, you may need to change the dose or type of medication taken before or after your operation. You should discuss with your doctor or pharmacist. Some bariatric centres recommend that medication be changed to chewable, liquid, dissolvable forms whilst on the liquid/pureed stage of the diet. If you take a number of tablets together in the early stages after surgery, this may fill up the new stomach/pouch with medication and there will be no space for food or fluid.

Childcare and Dependents

If you have a young family and/or care for others, you will need to consider and plan on having some help, whilst you are in hospital and also recovering from your operation.

During the recovery phase of your operation, you will have some pain, soreness, and fatigue as your body recovers from the surgery. You may find it painful to lift and carry children or support dependent adults. It is usually advisable to avoid carrying, lifting or pushing heavy objects until your wounds have fully healed, which is usually three to four weeks after surgery. This is to avoid bleeding or developing hernias around the port (wound) sites.

If you have a pet such as a dog or cat, you may need to make alternative arrangements for them to be cared for during your hospital stay and possibly in the early stages of recovery.

Driving

It is advised that you do not drive for up to 3 weeks after having abdominal surgery. You should check this with your motor insurance company before you have your operation, as they may invalidate your insurance if you drive too soon after having surgery. You will need to arrange for someone to come and collect you once you can go home after your operation.

Work

It is up to you whether or not you tell your work colleagues, but in most cases it may be advisable to tell your boss of your plans. Some employers may be willing to let you take time off as sick leave; others may make you take annual leave during your recovery. You should speak to them or your Human Resources Department to find out more information. Depending on how fast you recover and the level of physical activity included in your job, you are likely to require at least 2-4 weeks off work after your surgery.

What to Bring into Hospital

During your hospital stay you will need to consider taking the following in a small bag or small, portable suitcase. Leave any valuables such as jewellery at home.

- All your medication
- Dressing gown
- Nightie or pyjamas or T-shirt and shorts
- Slippers
- Socks
- Underwear
- Loose fitting clothes for when you go home
- Small amount of money
- Vitamin and mineral supplements
- Toiletry bag, including soap, face and body wash, toothpaste, toothbrush, shampoo, moisturising lotion, hairbrush, deodorant
- Towel

- Baby wipes
- Mobile phone and charger
- Magazines, book or tablet
- Some previous patients recommend a small pillow to place under your seatbelt for the journey home

Support Groups and Internet Forums

Most bariatric centres will have patient support groups for people who are thinking about or have had bariatric surgery. *Research has shown that people who attend support groups have better long-term weight-loss compared to those that do not attend.*

Support groups and forums are a useful way of sharing experiences and buddying up with others. Support groups can also be accessed via the Internet. It is important to find a support group or Internet forum that suits your needs. If people who attend the groups or Internet forums are from different centres, they may have different experiences and information to share.

When looking for a support group or Internet forum consider: -

- Is the support group or forum for anyone who has had bariatric surgery or is the group or forum only for people who have had bariatric surgery at one bariatric centre?
- Who runs the group or forum? Is it a patient or the dietitian or nurse from the centre you had your surgery?

- How often does the group meet?
- How long are the group meetings?
- Does the group have education sessions and guest speakers?
- How many people attend the group?
- Can family and friends attend?
- Do you need to book a place to attend the group?
- Is the location, accessibility and parking convenient to you?
- Is the support group discussion confidential?
- Who manages the group or Internet forum to ensure that the information provided and shared by other patients is accurate?

Be mindful that there will always be people who do not always tell the full truth or may exaggerate their experiences and weight loss.

Internet patient forums particularly can be misleading, with people posting their personal stories, thoughts, advice and ideas, which may not always be true. Choose a forum that is actively monitored, checked for accuracy and also removes inappropriate postings. Your bariatric centre should be able to recommended suitable websites and forums.

Whilst the Internet provides a wealth of information about bariatric surgery, there is also a lot of misinformation out there. Remember to follow the advice provided from your bariatric centre and if you are unsure about anything you have read on the Internet or have been told by another patient, then contact your bariatric surgery centre for advice.

Conclusion

Preparing for bariatric surgery is essential to help you make positive dietary and lifestyle changes for the long-term. By having the support network that is right for you before bariatric surgery, it will help with your recovery and ensure that you maintain the appropriate dietary and lifestyle changes required for long-term successful weight loss.

Chapter 7
What Happens Before, During and After Weight-Loss Surgery?

Before Surgery

Once you have selected your surgeon, you need to make an appointment to see him or her. Sometimes you will see the surgeon first and in some cases you will be seen initially by a dietitian or specialist nurse, and then by the surgeon.

The surgeon (or other members of the team) will ask you many questions about your weight, how long you have been overweight and why you think that you are overweight. They will ask you about your dietary habits and where you think you may have been going wrong. You will be asked about your general health and any medical problems that you may have; for example, they will ask if you suffer from diabetes, high blood pressure, breathing problems or heart disease. The surgeon will need to know about any medications that you are taking and any allergies that you have. You may be asked about whether you smoke or drink alcohol. You will be asked about whether or not you want surgery and, if so, which operation you prefer.

The surgeon (or others) will explain all the different surgical options to you, including any risks, potential complications, and expected weight loss of each procedure. Once you decided upon which operation you wish to undergo, you may be asked to sign a consent form (or this may be done when you come in for the operation). You will then be given a date and time to come in for your surgery.

Having organised a date for your admission to hospital, you may also be offered an appointment for a pre-operative assessment. In some cases this may be done at the same time as your initial consultation, but in most cases will involve another visit to the pre-assessment clinic. In selected cases, this may be done over the telephone to save you another visit to the hospital.

During the Hospital Stay

On the day of your operation, you will need to attend the hospital at the allotted time. You will need to bring nightwear and toiletries for however long you are expected to stay in hospital (usually one to three days, depending what operation you are having). You will be seen before the operation by both the surgeon and the anaesthetist, who will go through the procedure again with you and may ask you some further questions. If you have not already done so in the clinic, you will be asked to sign a consent form at this stage.

When you go to theatre for your operation, you will usually walk or be wheeled on your bed into the anaesthetic room, where you will be asked to lie on a trolley or bed. Sometimes you may be asked to lie on the actual operating table, which will later be wheeled into theatre. The anaesthetist will place a little plastic cannula (tube) into a vein usually in the back of the hand or at the front of the elbow joint. You will be put to sleep with an injection into this cannula. Sometimes you may be asked to breathe some oxygen from a mask over your nose and mouth before going to sleep.

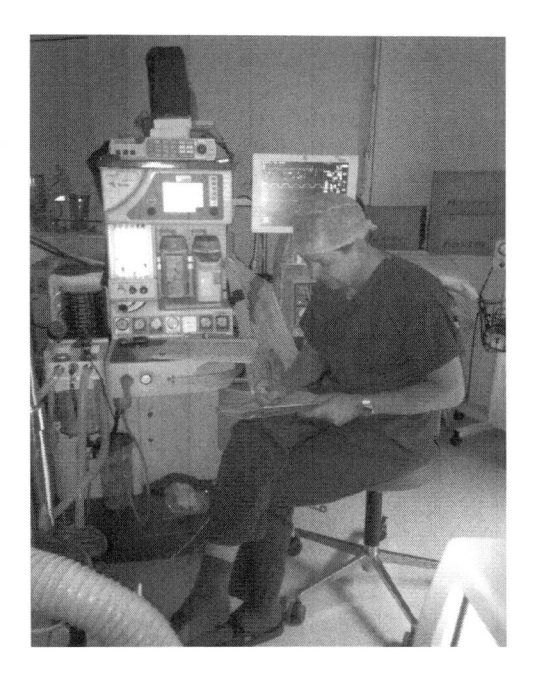

Bariatric anaesthetist

Once you are asleep you will be taken into theatre for your operation. Depending on the procedure, this may take anywhere from 20 minutes to a couple of hours. You may also have a urinary catheter (tube in your bladder to help you urinate) placed whilst you are asleep.

Once the procedure is complete, you will be woken up, usually in a sitting position in bed whilst still in theatre. Once you are awake and able to breathe for yourself, you will be taken to the theatre recovery room, where you will remain for a short while until ready to be returned to your room on the ward. Sometimes you will go back to the room you were in beforehand and sometimes you may go the high-dependency or critical-care unit for either a few hours or overnight, until you are well enough to return to the normal ward.

When you wake up, you will have an intravenous infusion (drip), through which you will be given fluids until you are able to drink normally. The amount you are allowed to drink will depend on the procedure that you have had performed. If you have had a laparoscopic gastric band operation, you will normally be allowed to drink freely almost immediately. If you have had a bigger procedure, such as a laparoscopic gastric bypass or laparoscopic sleeve gastrectomy, then you will usually be allowed small sips every hour on the day of your surgery, followed by free fluids the following day.

If you have had a urinary catheter placed then you will not need to worry about going to the toilet, as you will automatically pass water into the catheter bag. This will normally stay in place for the first night and is usually removed the following morning. A catheter is normally only placed for the bigger procedures and is rarely used with a gastric band.

This type of surgery, being laparoscopic ("key hole"), is not usually too painful and minimal pain relief is required. However, any pain relief that you do require, will all be sorted for you by the anaesthetist. You will normally have been given adequate pain relief in theatre, which should last for a period of time post-operatively. Sometimes all that will be required is oral analgesia and in other cases you may need infusions into the drip, but you should not expect to be in too much pain. Some patients complain of "wind pain" after the surgery and occasionally, with laparoscopic surgery, you may experience shoulder-tip pain. Both of these types of pain are short lived and usually settle within 24-48 hours of the operation.

After Surgery

Once you have recovered sufficiently, you will be allowed home. For a laparoscopic gastric band this is usually the following morning (or in some cases later on the day of surgery) and for the larger procedures, such as laparoscopic gastric bypass and laparoscopic sleeve gastrectomy, you will usually need to stay in hospital for two (occasionally three) nights.

One of the risks of any surgery (not just weight-loss surgery) is blood clots (deep venous thrombosis or DVT), which rarely can lead to a pulmonary embolism or PE (clot in the lungs). This can be a serious complication (even fatal in rare circumstances) and so every possible measure is taken to reduce this risk. Three measures are normally employed to counteract this problem. You will normally be issued with anti-embolism (TED) stockings, which you will need to put on before the operation and wear throughout your hospital stay and for a period of time after discharge (usually about six weeks). During the operation itself, special leggings will placed around your calves, which will provide intermittent calf compression (but you will be unaware of this). Very occasionally you may wake up in the recovery room still wearing these if the surgical team deem it necessary. The third measure that will be taken to reduce the risk of blood clotting is that you will be given injections under the skin. The needle used is tiny and this injection is relatively painless. In most circumstances you will need to continue these injections for a period of time (usually 10-28 days) after you go home. These are very easy to administer and most patients are able to administer these themselves (with a little training from the nursing staff whilst in hospital).

Nowadays, in the vast majority of cases, weight-loss surgery is performed laparoscopically (keyhole) and so the recovery is quicker. After gastric band surgery, you will normally need only a few days to recover and you should be fully recovered within one to two weeks. Most people are able to return to work after seven to ten days. The same will usually apply to driving. After a sleeve gastrectomy or gastric bypass, it may take a little longer to recover, but again, most people are able to return to work and drive within three to six weeks.

If you have had a laparoscopic gastric band, this will need to be adjusted from time to time. Gastric band adjustments are performed by the insertion of a (Huber) needle through the skin and into the "port" of the gastric band and the injection or removal of fluid, usually saline (salt water) into the gastric band. Injection of fluid will tighten the band (so that you are able to eat less) and removal of fluid will loosen the gastric band (so that you can eat more). This can be performed either by the doctor or nurse in the clinic room or in the x-ray department (where sometimes you may be asked to drink some fluid to assess the tightness of the gastric band). If necessary, this can be performed after the injection of some local anaesthetic. The first gastric band fill is usually carried out six weeks after the gastric band operation. Some people may only ever need one gastric band fill. Other people may need several adjustments to get an appropriate restriction.

After weight-loss surgery, all people are recommended to take oral daily multivitamin and mineral supplements for life. People who have a gastric bypass, sleeve gastrectomy, BPD +/-DS are recommended to have vitamin B12 injections once every three months for life.

It is important that people are seen regularly for post-surgical follow-up. The frequency of follow-up will depend on what operation has been performed and will vary from hospital to hospital. Most patients will be seen after about a month or so to see how they are getting on and then at various time intervals thereafter. The length of follow-up will also vary between centres but it is usually for one to three years.

Chapter 8

Complications or Problems after Weight-Loss Surgery

Bariatric surgery is very effective and successful, but like any operation, may cause complications. In the UK, there is a very low rate of complications, but they do still exist. It is important to make sure you understand what complications may happen, before you make the choice whether or not to have surgery. If you have any questions after reading this chapter, you should talk to your GP, surgeon, dietician, or you can find more information on the **simply**bariatrics.com website.

Complications from weight-loss surgery can be split into three categories:

- **General**- these can occur with ANY large operation, not just weight-loss surgery
- **Early**- meaning they occur within the first 30 days after surgery
- **Late** – these occur after the first 30 days, and can be years later

We will describe the general complications, and then the early and late complications for each of the common weight loss procedures performed in the UK, the gastric balloon, gastric band, sleeve gastrectomy and gastric bypass. We will also discuss the biliopancreatic diversion and duodenal switch, which are less commonly performed, because these may be associated with more complications. Most of the figures quoted in this chapter have been taken from the UK's NBSR (National Bariatric Surgery Registry) report, although figures will vary between countries. You should check with your local hospital or doctor to find out the complication rates for your bariatric team.

Information about the other weight loss procedures such as gastric plication, Endobarrier and POSE can be found on the simply*bariatrics*.com website.

General Complications

For the majority of procedures (except the gastric balloon and the Endobarrier), you need a general anaesthetic. Although general anaesthetics are very safe these days, there are still small risks, especially if you already have health problems. Before you undergo an anaesthetic, you will be given a pre-assessment appointment where they will do tests on your heart and possibly lungs, and take some blood tests. These make sure you are fit enough to undergo an anaesthetic. The anaesthetist will also see you and he will discuss the anaesthetic with you.

The most serious risks of the anaesthetic are from the possibility of a reaction to the drugs, which the anaesthetist will use to put you to sleep, and to keep your body systems working properly whilst the surgeon does the operation. If you have any known allergies, you should tell the surgeon and anaesthetist before the operation.

The biggest risks of the operation are of having a heart attack or stroke whilst you are under the anaesthetic. This is rare, but if you are very obese, your heart is already under strain and this increases the risk slightly. Around 0.03 percent of people (3 in 10 000) will have a heart attack or stroke after bariatric surgery.

Another potentially serious complication is getting a blood clot in the legs, which can travel to the lungs, causing a pulmonary embolism. You will be given injections and stockings to wear to try and avoid this. Approximately 0.04 percent of people (4 out of every 10 000) will get a pulmonary embolus (PE) and 0.03 percent (3 in 10 000) will develop Deep Vein Thrombosis (DVT). These numbers are much smaller than the risks for other types of elective surgery; for example, knee or hip replacements.

There is a mortality (death) risk with bariatric surgery. This risk is extremely small (1-2 people out of every 1000 people), and is much lower than for many other types of surgery, but it does exist.

Other complications that can occur with any operation include:

- Chest infections (around 0.2 percent or 2 in 1000)
- Wound infections (around 0.2 percent or 2 in 1000)
- On-going/persistent pain (rare)
- Significant scarring (rare)
- Constipation (uncommon)

All of the common bariatric operations are performed laparoscopically (keyhole), unless there are specific reasons for not doing the surgery this way. The surgeon will explain this to you if the surgery cannot be done laparoscopically. In order to do an operation via keyhole, the surgeon needs to make four, five, or six small holes in your abdominal wall. Any of these wounds can bleed after surgery, sometimes quite a lot. This can be known as a "port site haematoma" (meaning collection of blood at the port site). In most cases this will stop without help, but occasionally you need to have surgery to stop the bleeding.

Another problem that can happen, sometimes many years after surgery, is developing a small hernia in one of the wounds. This might also need surgery in the future, if it becomes painful or causes problems. This usually occurs in less than one percent of people.

Early Complications

These are the complications that can happen either during the operation itself, or in the first 30 days after surgery.

Gastric Balloon:

The main risks associated with having the gastric balloon are related to the camera procedure used to place or remove the balloon. There is a small risk of the camera pushing through the wall of the oesophagus or stomach, known as a perforation. In this case, you would need an operation to fix it. The general risk of this is one in 1500 people.

Other risks of endoscopy include a sore throat, and a very small risk of bleeding if the veins in your stomach or oesophagus are very large. There have been cases where a gastric balloon has been inflated in the oesophagus. Although rare, you would need an operation to fix this.

The balloon can leak. You would know because the fluid in the balloon would turn your urine blue. If this were to occur, it is not an emergency, but you should contact your bariatric team.

Gastric Band:

During the operation itself, the surgeon has to cut some of the tissues surrounding your stomach in order to be able to fit the band. This can cause some bleeding, which can usually be stopped fairly easily.

Very rarely, the surgeon may need to open your abdomen in order to be able to stop this bleeding. Risk of significant bleeding after gastric banding is around 0.09 percent (nine people in every 10 000).

The liver can often be very large (which is why people go on a pre-operative liver-shrinkage diet), and this can sometimes prevent the surgeon from being able to do the operation. The liver contains a large blood supply, and if it gets damaged during surgery, it can bleed heavily.

Rarely, the gastric band can be put in the wrong place, especially if there is a lot of fat within the abdomen itself, as the stomach has a large fat pad on the front. It has been known for the gastric band to be placed around this fat pad, not the stomach. This is not a major problem, and can usually be fixed with another operation. Also there is a very small risk of damage to the stomach.

Sleeve Gastrectomy:

Sleeve gastrectomy surgery is a longer operation. The main complications that can occur in the first few days after surgery are rare, but can be serious, and may mean you need another operation. However, it is rare to get late complications, so usually once you have recovered from the operation, it is unlikely you will experience any other major problems.

When the surgeon staples along the length of your stomach, this is like stapling thick sheets of paper together, and these staples can sometimes come apart, causing a leak of fluid and stomach acid into the abdomen. This means that anything you eat or drink also escapes from the stomach into the abdomen. In this case, it often takes an operation to fix it, although sometimes placing a tube down your nose and stopping you from eating or drinking can allow it to heal itself over a few days.

This join can also bleed, and if it bleeds enough, you may need a blood transfusion. Most of the time, this bleeding will stop on its own. The surgeon uses a special glue to help prevent this. Significant bleeding or leaking occurs in 0.6-1.3% of surgery patients.

Gastric Bypass:

Gastric bypass surgery is also a longer operation. The main operative complications that can occur are similar to the sleeve gastrectomy. When the surgeon joins the bowel to the stomach, or the bowel to the bowel, they either use a stapling device or stitch the tissues together. This is like joining two tubes together, and this join can sometimes leak. This is known as an 'anastomotic leak'. In this case, it often takes an operation to fix it.

These joins can also bleed, and if they bleed enough, you may need a blood transfusion or further surgery. Most of the time, this bleeding will stop on its own. Like the sleeve gastrectomy, leaks or bleeds occur in less than two out of every 100 people (0.6 percent leaks and 1.2 percent bleed).

Biliopancreatic diversion/duodenal switch (BPD/DS):

The BPD +/-DS is not routinely performed in the UK, because it is associated with a greater number of complications. BPD +/-DS surgery is a larger operation. Similarly to the gastric bypass, when the surgeon staples your stomach and bowel, the staples can come apart causing an 'anastomotic leak'. These joins can also bleed, and if they bleed enough, you may need a blood transfusion. Most of the time, this bleeding will stop on its own.

Late Complications

These complications can occur any time after surgery, in some cases, many years later. Late complications only occur with the gastric band, sleeve gastrectomy, gastric bypass and biliopancreatic diversion/duodenal switch, as these operations are designed to last lifelong (although the gastric band can be removed if necessary).

Gastric Balloon:

The balloon only stays in for six months, so the chances of developing late complications are rare. It is important to get the balloon removed after six months, as this is its life expectancy and the rubber can become damaged by the acid in your stomach.

Although the balloon needs removal after six months, sometimes the doctor is unable to remove it. This is more common if the balloon has leaked and it has passed out of the stomach. Sometimes the balloon can pass down the small bowel and get stuck. Occasionally, this may cause a blockage and you may need another procedure, either a camera up from the bottom end or an operation, to remove it.

Gastric Band:

The main risks of gastric band surgery occur late after the surgery, sometimes years later. Although they can happen in the first 30 days, they are more common months or years after surgery.

Gastric band slippage: the gastric band should sit around the top of the stomach, causing a small pouch above it. Sometimes the gastric band can slip upwards, making this pouch much smaller than it should be which causes pain, heartburn, and can make you vomit frequently. Slippage is diagnosed with a test called a contrast swallow.

You will be asked to drink a chalky fluid called barium, and then X-rays are taken. The position of the gastric band can be seen on this X-ray. Usually, this test is only performed if you are experiencing these symptoms. Gastric band slippage can be detected on an X-ray even if there are no symptoms. However, around five to ten percent of people with a gastric band (less than 5-10 in 100) will have symptoms caused by band slippage.

Once a band slippage is diagnosed, taking the fluid out of the band can often treat it, and make the gastric band move back into the correct position. However, in some cases this does not happen, and the gastric band needs repositioning, which requires an operation, similar to your original one. Sometimes the gastric band cannot be repositioned, and in these cases, it may need removal.

Gastric band erosion: the gastric band can erode into the stomach (go through the wall) and this unfortunately means it has to be removed. In this case, it cannot be replaced, as it will have caused a lot of scar tissue on your stomach. This is rare, and usually occurs in 0-1 percent out of every 100 people.

The gastric band can absorb or lose fluid: sometimes the gastric band will draw in fluid spontaneously, making it too tight and requiring it be loosened. Alternatively, the gastric band can slowly leak fluid, meaning that you need to get it tightened more often. Occasionally this is because there is a small hole in the gastric band or the gastric band tubing. It may take another operation to fix or replace the gastric band.

Gastric band port: some people can experience problems with the gastric band port, which is usually placed below the ribs on the left side of the abdominal wall, just underneath the skin. Sometimes this port can become infected, especially if the skin is not cleaned properly before fluid is injected into it. The port can however become infected even if everything is cleaned properly, because it is a foreign body. If you get a port infection, you might notice pain or redness over the port site. Occasionally, this can be managed with antibiotics, however in many cases the port may need to be removed. Usually this can be replaced at a later date, but it does mean that your gastric band might not work whilst there is no port.

The port can also erode through the skin, and again, if this happens it will need to be removed. In most cases the port can be replaced at a later date, but sometimes these complications mean that the gastric band no longer works, as the fluid will leak out. In many centres, the gastric band fills are done by feeling for the port and injecting it with fluid. Some bariatric centres will undertake most of their band fills using X-rays; this is up to the centre.

If the port cannot be identified, the radiologist can use an ultrasound machine to see where the port is, and access it to adjust your gastric band. An ultrasound does not require any X-rays and is completely safe. Occasionally the port cannot be accessed, especially if it has flipped over, and you need a small operation to fix it back into its proper place. Around one percent (1 in 100) of people may have one of the above problems with their port or port tubing.

Sleeve Gastrectomy:

Long-term (or 'late') complications following the sleeve gastrectomy are rare, but occasionally do happen.

Strictures (narrowing): the staple line made in the stomach during the operation heals in the first couple of weeks after surgery, but sometimes it can over-heal, causing a narrowing, which is known as a stricture. In this case, it may be difficult to eat properly, and patients can experience pain, vomiting, and acid reflux. If the narrowing is very tight, this stricture may need stretching (dilatation) using an endoscopy and a balloon. This is usually only needed once to resolve this problem. However, some people may need this procedure repeating a number of times. Strictures are usually seen in around five percent (5 in 100) of people.

Ulceration: occasionally, people can develop ulcers in their remaining stomach because of the acid secreted by the stomach. Most of the time, this can be treated with medication. Some bariatric centres will recommend antacid medication for the first few months after surgery to help prevent ulceration. Your doctor may recommend you avoid non-steroidal anti-inflammatory drugs (NSAIDs) life long to help prevent ulceration. Ulceration has been seen in approximately five percent (5 in 100) of people.

Nutritional deficiencies: vitamin and mineral deficiencies can occur in the long-term. The most common deficiencies are iron, calcium, vitamin D, vitamin B12 and folic acid. These are more common if you do not take a complete A-Z multi vitamin and mineral supplement on a daily basis and eat a low nutritional value diet.

Gastric Bypass:

Long-term (or 'late') complications following the gastric bypass are rare, but do occasionally happen.

Strictures (narrowing) - similarly to the sleeve gastrectomy, the join between the stomach and the bowel, or the join between the two loops of small bowel can over-heal. This is again known as a stricture. This stricture may need stretching, sometimes a number of times, with a camera test and a balloon. This can occur in up to 5 percent (5 in 100) of people.

Fistula - in very rare cases, a communication between the stomach (which although is not used for eating, is left in the abdomen so it can still secrete hormones) and the small bowel occurs. This is known as a 'fistula'. It may cause heartburn or vomiting, or can sometimes cause you to put weight back on.

Ulceration - like following the sleeve gastrectomy, people can develop ulcers in their stomach pouch or at one of the joins in the bowel because of the digestive juices. Most of the time, this can be treated with medication. Some bariatric centres will recommend antacid medication for the first few months after surgery to help prevent ulceration. You may be recommended by your centre to avoid non-steroidal anti-inflammatory drugs (NSAIDs) life long to help prevent ulceration. Ulceration has been seen in approximately 5 percent (5 in 100) of people.

Nutritional deficiencies - vitamin and mineral deficiencies can occur in the long-term. The most common deficiencies are iron, calcium, vitamin D, vitamin B12 and folic acid. These are more common if you do not take a complete A-Z multi vitamin and mineral supplement on a daily basis and eat a low nutritional value diet.

Biliopancreatic diversion/duodenal switch (BPD +/-DS):

The BPD/DS is reserved for people who have a greater amount of excess body weight to lose or need to lose more weight following other types of surgery (mainly after the gastric bypass or sleeve gastrectomy).

Nutritional deficiencies - the major complication that occurs after a BPD +/-DS is malabsorption. This means that you cannot absorb as much in the way of protein. You may not absorb the vitamins and minerals as effectively that your body needs to keep you healthy. This can lead to health problems, even if you take all your multivitamins and mineral supplements. So it is important to ensure that you have your vitamin and mineral blood levels checked regularly.

Diarrhoea - this side effect is also a common problem, particularly after the BPD +/-DS surgery. It is often because you do not absorb as much food and fluid because your bowel is deliberately made shorter by the surgery. If you eat a high fat diet, you may find the diarrhoea also smells and is difficult to flush away.

Dumping syndrome - dumping syndrome also causes diarrhoea. This is when high sugar foods enter the small bowel too quickly, and it draws a lot of water into the bowel with it. This then passes quickly through your system and causes diarrhoea. Some people report that their flatus (wind) also smells very bad which can be distressing and uncontrollable.

Excessive weight loss - sometimes, people lose too much weight, or cannot absorb enough protein, vitamins and minerals following this operation. This can mean there is a need for special feeding through the veins. This is called parenteral nutrition and may be required in the long term if your body does not adjust to the dietary advice and medication advised.

Other Effects of Bariatric Surgery

Loose Skin

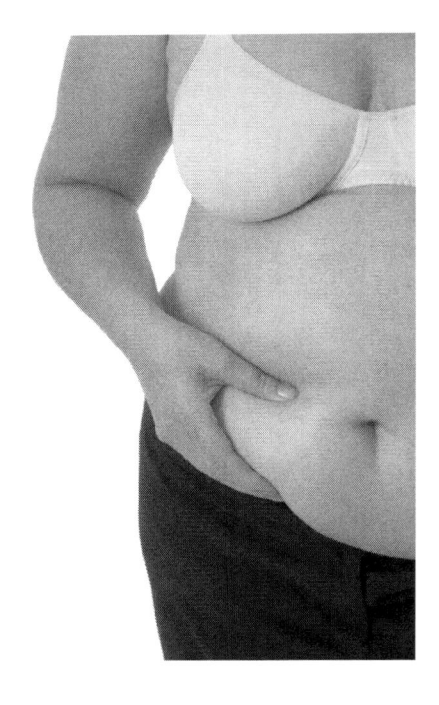

Patients may be left with loose skin.

Although not a complication, something that can cause people problems is loose skin. Loose skin is a common problem after bariatric surgery. The more weight you have to lose, the higher the chances of getting loose skin become. Some people say that regular exercise, massage, or moisturising their skin helps to minimise the amount of loose skin they have, but this does not always work. In most cases, there is nothing that can be done other than getting plastic surgery to remove it. *It is very unlikely that you will be able to get state funded skin removal surgery*, because it does not usually cause health problems - it is done for cosmetic reasons. In most cases, if you want skin surgery, you will have to pay for it privately. It is usually a good idea to wait until you have stopped losing weight and have maintained it for at least 6 months to a year before considering surgery, or you may lose more weight and end up with even more loose skin. In this chapter, we have described the **physical** complications that can occur after bariatric surgery. We have not discussed the psychological problems that some people find occur. These include:

- An increase in depression or anxiety, particularly in people who were depressed or anxious before surgery.
- Issues around sexuality. Some people have been sexually abused in the past, and losing weight can make them feel very vulnerable.

- Change to relationships, particularly with partners. If someone has been overweight for a long time, and then loses a lot of weight, it can cause a change in their relationship when they cannot eat as much as before, or the partner can become jealous if they start looking more attractive and want to socialise more than they did before.
- Addiction transference. Many people who have been overweight are so because they are addicted to food. After surgery, they can no longer eat as much, so their addiction to food transfers to things like alcohol, drugs or gambling, exercise or shopping, for example.

Body dysmorphia causes people to still see themselves as bigger, even if they are a healthy size. This can cause psychological problems, or they might not like the way their new body looks and this can be distressing.

If you are worried about any of these psychological issues, you should talk to your GP, dietician or surgeon before you consider surgery. More information can be found on the **simply**bariatrics.com website.

When to Seek Urgent Help after Weight-Loss Surgery?

There are a number of "red flag" symptoms, which, if you experience them, you should seek help from your family doctor, bariatric team or emergency department in the hospital:

Emergency hospital advice:

- Vomiting blood
- Abdominal pain not controlled with simple pain killers (those given to you by the hospital)
- Inability to swallow *any* food or liquid
- Painful, discoloured lumps that you cannot push flat in any of your wound sites or scars

Bariatric team or family doctor:

- Difficulty with swallowing (but able to swallow liquids)
- Mild abdominal pain
- Unexplained vomiting after eating food
- Symptoms of dumping syndrome
- Pain/ redness/ swelling of your gastric band port
- Lumps that come and go in your wound sites or scars
- Hair loss

Chapter 9
Care and Recovery after Bariatric Surgery

Follow-up by the Bariatric Team

It is extremely important that a plan is arranged before your discharge for an appropriate follow-up by your bariatric team. Ensure you clearly know the date, time, and venue of your next follow-up appointment. After all bariatric surgical procedures, follow-up should be life long. Usually the first two years you will be followed-up by the surgical team and thereafter followed up by your family doctor.

Ensure that you communicate with your team whether you are able to follow the appropriate dietary stages as directed by your dietitian. It is important to let the team know if you have any of the following: nausea, vomiting, heartburn, constipation, dumping syndrome, excessive hair loss, or any symptoms that you are uncomfortable with.

**Ten Points to Remember
During Follow-Up Consultations**

1. Explain, in detail, any problems you have encountered after discharge.
2. Discuss the quantity and textures of food and fluids you have consumed.
3. If you have a band, you may have a band fill, if appropriate.
4. Discuss about vitamin/mineral supplements and doses.
5. Ensure you have all the necessary investigations and discuss results of their outcomes.
6. Seek help if you have any psychological or social issues, do not delay.
7. Get yourself weighed and have weight-loss and BMI calculated.
8. Do not forget to discuss return to work, exercise, sex, and relationships.
9. Discuss any associated medical conditions you have and if medications need to be changed/reduced with weight-loss.
10. Finally agree on the date/time of your next consultation.

Purely restrictive procedures like gastric band or sleeve gastrectomy usually cause digestive symptoms, food intolerance, altered eating behaviour or reflux. However, gastric bypass or Biliopancreatic diversion, which results in malabsorption, may result in iron deficiency and increased risk of calcium, vitamin D and vitamin B12 deficiencies. In addition to the usual blood tests like haemoglobin, full blood count, kidney function, liver function, bone profile,

Vitamin B12, your doctor may also request tests like zinc, selenium, parathyroid hormone (PTH), if required in addition to the regular blood tests.

Finally, it is important to remember that if you do not feel well, do not wait for the next appointment, and seek medical help immediately.

Family and Friends

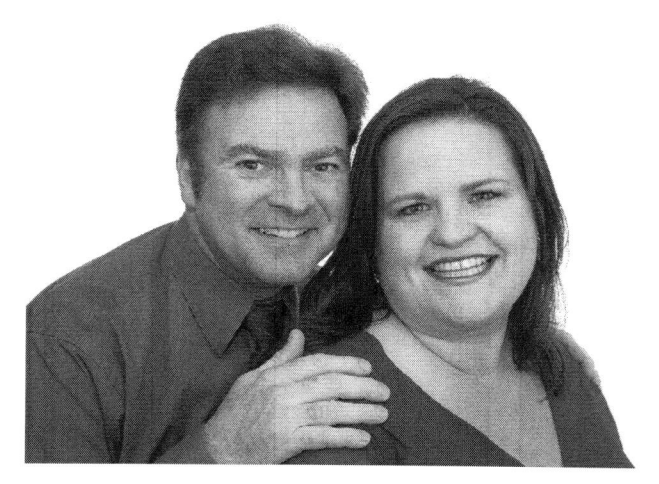

Family and friends

You may need support from your friends and family both before and after surgery to have safe, successful, long-term weight loss. Having weight-loss surgery is a personal decision, but it helps to ensure that you have people who you can talk to, as surgery is life-changing. Some people join local or Internet-based support groups or buddy up with people who had surgery at the same time as they did.

Many people find that their life changes significantly after surgery, particularly from the health benefits they have felt from the weight loss they have achieved. People tend to be more socially active and want to go out and do the things that they felt they could not or were unable to do before surgery.

This can sometimes put a strain on some relationships. It may be that you cannot eat the same foods as your friends and family want to eat or family members still want to give you larger portions of food. Talking to the people close to you, and making sure they understand how the surgery is likely to change your and their lives is important. Before surgery, you may want your partner, or a friend, to attend your clinic appointments with you so that they understand what your weight-loss journey may be. Sometimes, they will help by changing their lifestyle; this extra support can help make sure you follow your dietary and lifestyle advice.

Some people choose not to tell their friends or family about their plans for bariatric surgery. This decision is up to you and how you feel. However, you may find people asking you about your weight loss and possible changes in diet. It is a good idea to think about what you will tell them before you have your operation.

Work

It may take a few weeks before you are ready to go back to work after surgery. The amount of time this takes depends on which operation you have and your health.

It is always a good idea to warn your employers that you will be taking time off work. This way, they can find people to cover your work during your absence. Most employers would prefer to be given advance notice of your absence, rather than finding out after you've had surgery.

In most cases, especially if you are having weight-loss surgery to improve your health, employers will be supportive of your decision to have an operation, and will do what they can to make getting time off work as easy as possible. If you do not feel comfortable talking to your manager about your surgery, you could try your human resources department and ask for advice.

Honesty with people is usually the best policy!

Smoking and Alcohol

Any doctor or nurse will always advise that you stop smoking or drinking alcohol before surgery. Smoking increases the risk of having heart and lung problems during surgery, and increases the risk of most of the other complications (bleeding, blood clots, infections, poor healing, staple-line leaks, strictures etc.). In some hospitals, the surgeons will not operate on you if you cannot prove (with a breathing test) that you have quit smoking.

Drinking large amounts of alcohol causes liver damage and contributes to being obese—alcohol has a high calorie, low nutritional content. You are advised not to drink alcohol after surgery. The length of time you will be advised to avoid alcohol varies between procedures. Alcohol can be rapidly absorbed after bariatric surgery and it can affect your liver function, particularly with the expected weight loss.

Medications

In the first few weeks after surgery, you may find that some of your tablets are difficult to swallow, or you may fill up on your tablets and have no room for food. It is important to make sure that you are able to take all of your usual medications after surgery.

Your doctor or pharmacist can often advise you on alternative ways of taking your medications, i.e. whether your tablets can be crushed or dissolved. Some tablets cannot be crushed or dissolved (they lose their action if you do this) and therefore they will need to be changed to a liquid version.

In some cases, your doctor may have to change your tablets to other medications that you can take after surgery.

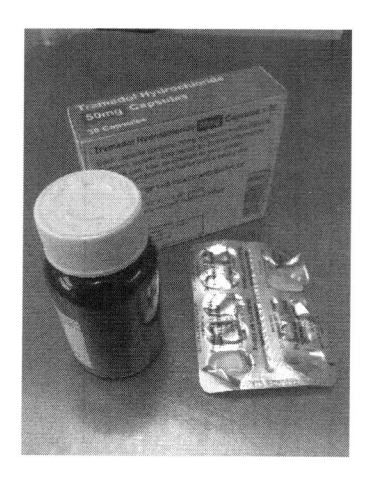

Medications

It is a good idea to speak to your doctor or pharmacist about temporarily changing your medication to alternative forms before you go for surgery, so you are ready and prepared for when you leave the hospital.

Overcoming Dumping Syndrome

Dumping syndrome is an unfortunate consequence of many types of bariatric surgery, especially the gastric bypass, sleeve gastrectomy, BPD and DS. Not everyone experiences dumping syndrome, but those that do can experience a number of side effects.

Dumping syndrome can be *early* or *late*.

Early dumping: This is due to food leaving the pouch/stomach and entering the small bowel too quickly. This food then draws a lot of fluid into the bowel. This tends to occur 15-30 minutes after a meal. Symptoms usually include abdominal pain, bloating, nausea or vomiting, dizziness, fainting and diarrhoea.

Late dumping: This is caused by the pancreas secreting large amounts of the hormone insulin in response to food entering the first part of the small bowel (duodenum). It tends to occur one to three hours after eating. Symptoms include dizziness, fainting, tremor, confusion, and weakness. Blood sugar may become low.

Most people with dumping syndrome find that certain foods, such as carbohydrates or sugars, are most likely to cause dumping syndrome, and avoidance of these foods can prevent symptoms. Eating small, but more frequent meals can also help. Unfortunately, there is no definite way to avoid this consequence of bariatric surgery, and you should be aware of these symptoms before you have any operation.

If you experience dumping syndrome, some things that can help include:

- Lie down

- Drink regular sips of water
- Put a cold wet towel on your forehead
- Avoid alcohol

Hair Loss

Hair loss is common after weight-loss operations, especially in the first few weeks and months due to the stress of surgery. In most cases, this will grow back.

After surgery, hair loss can sometimes be worse if the patient experiences any illnesses or traumas, if you have any hormonal imbalances, or with certain medications such as beta-blockers, vitamin A excesses, and blood-thinning medications (anti-coagulants). Lack of zinc, folate, biotin, and vitamin B6 can also contribute to hair loss.

In most cases, eating a healthy balanced diet and taking your daily multi-vitamins will help to avoid significant hair loss, or help your hair to grow back. If you find your hair loss is worse than expected, you should visit your family doctor or bariatric team for more advice.

Food Preparation Equipment

There are a few pieces of equipment that you may wish to consider buying or borrowing before surgery. By preparing before surgery, it should make recovery from your operation a little easier, particularly if you have already have made preparations for food after your surgery, before you have your surgery.

Food Blender: Initially after surgery, you will be on a liquid and pureed diet, which involves blending all of your food (see our "After Surgery" webpage). Using a blender is important to ensure that there are no lumps or bits in your food in the early stages after surgery. It is advised to blend and prepare food prior to your surgery, so that you have less food preparation and cooking whilst you are recovering from your surgery.

Ice cube trays: After bariatric surgery many people find that freezing portions of blended food into ice cube trays is very helpful. Initially after surgery, you will only be able to manage 2-3 tablespoons of blended/pureed food. Ice cube containers generally provide the correct size to pop the frozen pureed food and reheat as required. This will help prevent overestimating your portions sizes and reduce food wastage too.

Chapter 10
Physical Activity after Bariatric Surgery

This chapter provided by
Mohan Ramasamy, Specialist Weight Management Physiotherapist

Where do I start?

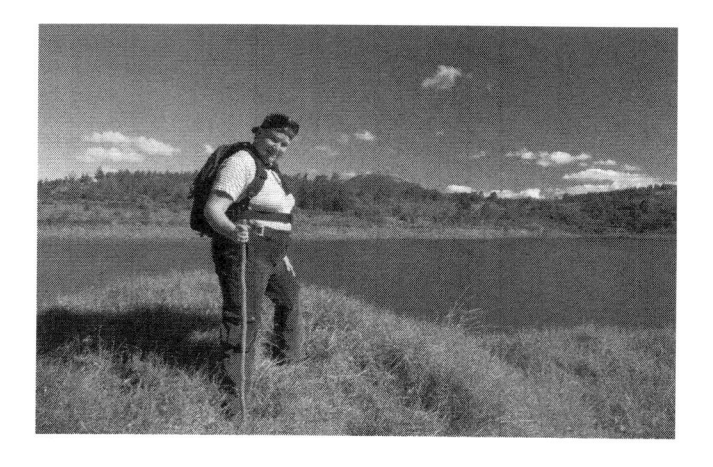

Exercise is an important part of weight loss and the success of your bariatric surgery. It should be done properly without overpowering your body. The recovery time after bariatric surgery and what activities are restricted during the healing process are the important things that need to be considered before you start any exercise programme. The type of surgery you have and your overall health status need to be taken into consideration before you start your regular physical activities. It may take eight weeks to get back to your pre-operative level. It is essential to develop a new routine of doing some physical activity as a part of your new lifestyle.

Type and intensity of exercises are very important within the first eight weeks following the surgery. After surgery, your body will get fewer calories because you will be eating less; so, it is important to focus on aerobic fat burning exercise as soon as possible in order to use your excess body fat as a fuel for your activities and prevent muscle loss. Otherwise your body tends to take energy from muscle protein in order to compensate for the reduced input energy; this way the body ends up losing muscle rather than body fat. Therefore it is good to start with gentle non-weight bearing, low impact aerobics and then gradually progress on to various intensity levels and type of exercises.

How much energy does your workout burn?

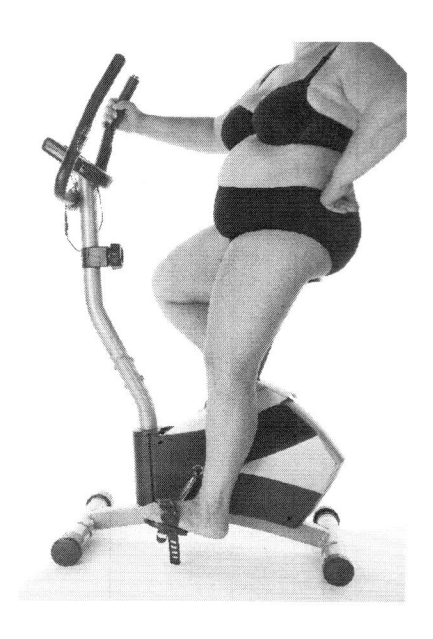

Metabolic equivalent, is a way of measuring the energy you have spent for your physical activities and use this simple formula to calculate how much energy you burned in your workout:

> Total Calories Burned = Duration of your physical activities in Minutes x { (MET x 3.5 x your weight in kg)/200}

(1 MET is equivalent to a metabolic rate consuming 3.5 millilitres of oxygen per kilogram of body weight per minute)

(1 MET is equivalent to a metabolic rate consuming 1 kilocalorie per kilogram of body weight per hour)

MET for Various Physical Activities

Light Intensity (<3 MET)

Sleeping	0.9
Riding in a car or bus	1.0
Lying quietly, sitting quietly	1.0
Reading, talking on telephone	1.5
Sitting, studying, note taking	1.8
Standing, walking at a very slow pace (less than 2 mph), playing musical instrument, light gardening, light office work, light use of hand tools (watch repair or micro-assembly, light assembly/repair); standing-light work (bartending, store clerk, assembling, filing), laundry, cooking, making bed	2.0
Walking at a slow pace (2 mph), walking downstairs, walking the dog, walking to neighbour's house or family's house for social reasons, walking from house to car or bus, light housekeeping, general cleaning, washing dishes, multiple household tasks all at once (light effort), ironing, shopping, pushing stroller with child, mild stretching, billiards game	2.5
Walking 2.5 mph, downhill	2.8

Moderate Intensity (3-6 MET)

Walking (2.5 mph), downstairs walking, standing doing light/moderate work (assemble/repair heavy parts, welding, auto repair, pack boxes for moving, etc.), patient care (as in nursing); driving heavy tractor, bus or truck, washing car or windows, moderately vigorous playing with children, sweeping outside house, picking fruit or vegetables, weight lifting (moderate effort), fishing general, bowling, loading / unloading a car, painting, paper hanging, scraping   3.0

Walking at a moderate pace (3 mph), weight lifting (moderate), leisurely canoeing or kayaking, walking on job (3 mph) in office - moderate speed, not carrying anything or carrying only light articles, home exercise(light or moderate effort, general), multiple household tasks all at once (moderate effort), vacuuming, mopping, scrubbing floors   3.5

Walking at a brisk pace (3.5 mph), dancing (moderately fast), leisurely bicycling <10 mph, raking lawn, planting shrubs, weeding garden, heavy yard work or gardening activities, masonry, moderately heavy lifting continuously, moderately heavy farm   4.0

work, multiple household tasks all at once (vigorous effort), water aerobics, playing with children (moderate), horseback riding

Slow swimming, golf (carrying clubs), dancing (disco, folk, line, country dancing), mowing lawn (hand mower)   4.5

Low impact aerobics, walking at a very brisk pace (4 mph), most doubles tennis, dancing (more rapid), some exercise apparatuses (elliptical trainer, stepper, stationary bike), Digging, spading, vigorous gardening, using heavy power tools; general gardening, Painting, carpentry, cleaning gutters, laying carpet, other vigorous activities, Chopping wood, playing cricket (batting, bowling)   5.0

Slow jogging (one mi every 13 to 14 min), ice or roller-skating, doubles tennis (if you run a lot)   6

Anaerobic activities (weight lifting vigorous – free weight, power lifting or body building, walking 3.5 mph uphill, swimming leisurely, hiking   6.5

Vigorous Intensity (> 6 MET)

Rowing, canoeing, kayaking vigorously, dancing (vigorous), jogging general, badminton   7

(competitive), high impact aerobics, tennis general, squash, racquetball	
Walking at 5 mph, climbing upstairs, bicycling general, water jogging, jogging in place, skiing downhill or cross country, heavy farming work, volleyball, basketball (competitive), running 5 mph	8
Football (competitive), Running cross country	9
Running 6 mph (10-minute mile), Jumping Rope, swimming laps fast	10
Swimming free style vigorous, bicycling stationary, very vigorous effort, HIIT (High Intensity Interval Training)	12.5
Running 8 mph (7.5-minute mile)	13.5
Running 10 mph (6-minute mile)	16

Exercise Protocol after Bariatric Surgery

During Hospital Stay:

Generally, it will take few days to recover enough to discharge from hospital after bariatric surgery, so during hospital stay, gentle walking is an ideal exercise to improve blood circulation throughout your body. Walk as much as possible, several times a day. It doesn't matter how long you walk; even if you walk a few minutes, it will still help your healing process.

First Week after Hospital Discharge

After you are discharged from hospital, you can start to walk around your home five to ten minutes at a time, several times in day. Walk on a flat, even surface until your doctor gives consent for uphill or downhill walking, as it puts more stress on your abdominal muscles. Avoid treadmill walking at this earlier stage, as it is too much exertion at this point. Try to walk each day bit further than previous day. You can gradually include an appropriate exercise programme into your daily routine, once you get consent from your doctor. It is crucial to increase your physical activity gradually, rather than doing too much too soon and harm yourself. During the healing process, avoid lifting more than 5 kg.

Initial Stage—Weeks 2 - 5

It's not safe to put more stress on healing abdominal muscles for the first six weeks. An abdominal hernia may happen if your surgical incision does not heal well; therefore, you should avoid any strenuous strengthening exercise for abdominal muscles, vigorous aerobic exercise, and fast brisk walking in first six weeks after surgery. Your exercise plan should be slow, gradual, and controlled. You can start with relaxed, gentle exercises in a standing or sitting position, at a slow pace.

Isometric Abdominal Exercise:

You can start with simple bed exercises without hurting abdominal muscles. Lie on your back with a pillow under your head to prevent over stretching of your abdominal muscles. Bend both knees, breathe gentle and slow, and gently pull your tummy in by tightening the abdominal muscle and holding it for three to ten seconds. Feel your lower back flat against the floor and then relax. Repeat this exercise three to five times, two to five times a day.

Gentle Exercise One:

Sit nice and tall in a chair or stand with your hands on your hips. Move your feet forward alternately by sliding one heel, along with your hand, following your foot. Repeat this five to ten times, twice a day.

Gentle Exercise Two:

Sit nice and tall in a chair or stand with your hands on your hips, then move one foot alternately backward and same time stretch both arms forward, repeat this five to ten times, twice in day.

Intermediate Stage— Week 6 - 13

At this point, you can add gentle strengthening exercise for your abdominal muscles and simple low-impact aerobics in a standing or sitting position. Discuss with your doctor and get consent before starting abdominal strengthening exercise.

Gentle Abdominal Exercise:

When you feel your abdominal muscles are less sore, lie on your back with both knees bent and feet flat on the bed or floor. Keep your hands on your thighs and slowly slide them towards your knees. Do not extend beyond your pain-free range. Hold this position for two to five seconds, and then slowly lie back down. Repeat this exercise five to ten times, two to five times a day.

Aerobic Exercise One:

March with your feet on the floor while sitting in a chair or standing. Punch your arms alternatively forward, repeating for about one minute, twice a day.

Aerobic Exercise Two:

Stand up or sit up straight in a chair, with your feet together and arms at your side. Move one foot sideways and make wider step along with pushing your hand backwards. Repeat for about one minute, twice a day.

Advanced Stage—Week 14 - 19

You can slowly increase your exercise session by adding more simple aerobics and gradually increasing your exercise intensity level by increasing your speed. Please avoid any high impact exercise such as jumping or related activities.

Example Exercises:

Marching on your feet on the floor and then slowly swing your arms forward and backward alternatively for one minute continuously like walking in place. If you need a rest because you feel breathless or experience leg tiredness, don't stop the exercise suddenly. Instead, slow down your speed or gently raise your heels up and down until you feel better, then carry on with the exercise.

Maintenance Stage—Week 20 and Beyond

You can add more abdominal strengthening exercises such as modified abdominal crunches. Focus on more aerobic activities, such as brisk walking, swimming, aquatic aerobics, cycling, and cardiovascular exercise by using equipment like a treadmill, cross-trainer, static bike, or rowing machine.

Long-Term Success:

If you want to continue your exercise programme for the long term, it is important to develop your own physical activity regimen based on your preferences and try it a little each day. You should include various types of exercise in to your workout such as aerobic, flexibility, strengthening, high-calories burning, and aquatic exercise.

Chapter 11
Sex and Relationships after Bariatric Surgery

Post-Surgical Sex Life

Many people ask how soon after bariatric surgery they can have sex. You can have sex as soon as you feel physically well and comfortable to do so. Ensure the wounds have all healed and you are feeling physically and mentally fine. Generally, most people resume sexual activity two to four weeks after weight-loss surgery. Consult your doctor or bariatric team if you are unsure. It is recommended that you use some form of barrier contraception to start with. As mentioned in the chapter on pregnancy, it is advisable to avoid pregnancy for 18 months after surgery so that all the changes that your body is undergoing do not affect your baby.

Take it easy! As you lose weight, your partner may feel benefits too from your weight loss and may want to try new positions with you, or increase the frequency of intercourse. Proceed gently, discuss how you feel with your partner, and take your time to adapt to your new body.

Obese men and women often feel under-confident and can have performance anxiety. They do not socialise as much and have a false belief that they are not sexually attractive.

Some women have an imbalance between their male and female hormones. This results in irregular menstrual periods and increased facial hair. Increased facial hair adds to their reduced confidence. Some obese women have a history of sexual abuse, which may have been the primary cause for weight gain. They feel they would be vulnerable to sexual attacks if they lose weight and look sexually attractive.

About 30 percent of morbidly obese men have some form of erectile dysfunction. The scrotum lies outside the body so that it is about two degrees centigrade cooler than the body temperature. This enables the testicles to function well. When a man is significantly obese, the fat cushions the testicles, warming them back up to normal body temperature. Also, excess fat tissue produces certain substances that prevent testosterone being converted to an active form.

Weight loss follows after weight-loss surgery. Even moderate weight loss can improve sexual function.

With weight loss there is:

1. Improved confidence

2. Improved body image

3. Less performance anxiety

4. Reduced facial hair in women

5. Regular periods with correction of hormonal imbalance

6. Scrotum lies away from the body, so is less than the body temperature and the testicles can function better

7. Increased availability of active form of testosterone

8. No hesitation on body positioning during intercourse

One study showed that women who had weight-loss surgery had an improvement in their sexual desire, arousal, lubrication, ability to achieve orgasm, and sexual satisfaction. This may be due in part to general improvement in quality of life and general well being.

Sexual function may not always improve with weight loss. Women who have had a history of sexual abuse do not seem to benefit as much from weight loss after bariatric surgery.

In some individuals, sexual desire and activity may, in fact, worsen after bariatric surgery. This may be due to distorted body image, identity problems, and disturbed relationships with existing partners. Most importantly, excess skin, especially the skin of the abdominal wall, which overhangs, makes them feel less attractive, and the overhanging skin can interfere with sexual activity.

This chapter deals with sex and relationship before and after surgery. During preparation for surgery, you should discuss sex and your relationship with your partner. You should have realistic expectations after surgery. Research shows that there is an improvement in sexual functioning after weight loss. This may be due to a number of factors including improvement in self-esteem, confidence and changes in your hormonal activity.

Post-Surgical Relationships

Sexual satisfaction and relationships are vital to your sense of well being and social functioning. Relationships change in several ways after weight-loss surgery. Your relationship with yourself, your family, your friends, and colleagues will change depending on how you feel and how other people see you.

Most people experience an increase in self-confidence. It has been reported that good relationships improve and not-so-good relationships may get worse. Excess skin may be upsetting and can affect your relationship. You may also find difficulty in socialising as you have changed your eating and drinking habits after surgery.

Often partners share their eating and drinking habits and following surgery your partner may find it difficult to adjust to the change. Eating together may have been the only bond between the partners and when this is disturbed, breakdown in relationship follows. It is therefore extremely important to discuss these issues with your partner or seek help from a counsellor.

You may notice that people will start to treat you differently; this in turn, may or may not be acceptable to your partner. Your partner may feel insecure and this may negatively influence your relationship. Divorce rates following bariatric surgery are very high.

You should talk to your family, friends, and your health care team before and after bariatric surgery. Seek help from your doctor if you are not able to adjust to the changes you encounter in different relationships.

Sex after bariatric surgery

Most people are conscious of their body and hence they do not have a normal sexual life. With weight loss your body image will improve, but more importantly you will be healthier and your confidence in performing should get better. It is extremely important to understand that sex does not have to equate to penetrative sexual intercourse.

Men who are overweight or obese have sexual problems due to performance anxiety and to some extent due to an alteration in hormonal balance. Weight loss after surgery improves hormones, but may not always improve performance. It is therefore important to understand that your ability to perform depends on you. Have a realistic goal. Discuss with your partner and do not aim for penetrative sexual intercourse to start with.

You can start to get intimate after surgery as soon as you feel better about yourself; however, give your body some time to recover after surgery before performing any penetrative sexual activity. A number of factors can lead to reduced desire to have sex or reduced ability to perform, even if you have the desire. Some of these are listed below:

- Past experience
- Medications
- Anxiety
- Low mood
- Unrealistic expectation
- Unable to find a suitable position

Follow these seven important steps to succeed in your sexual performance:

- Be open with your partner about your needs.
- Take it one step at a time.
- Be relaxed, set small goals.
- Plan a suitable atmosphere.
- Find the right place and time.
- Be intimate before you plan to have any sexual activity.
- Avoid excessive caffeine or alcohol.

Some people who have weight problems, have difficulty performing penetrative sexual intercourse; however, with change in position and a cooperative partner, this issue can be overcome. Here are a few suggestions for sex positions after bariatric surgery. As mentioned above, only attempt these if you feel well and have completely recovered from surgery.

Sex positions

No one sex position is better than another. You will need to work with your partner to find a suitable position. Working with your partner to increase intimacy and desire is more important than attempting penetrative intercourse. Again, position depends on the size of your partner. Some of the position listed below may help obese couples:

- Male dominant position
- Female on top

- Female on top, back to front
- Rear entry position
- X position
- Standing position
- T-square position

Make use of aids and pillows if required. Also, remember foreplay is more important than the actual act of performing sex.

Sexercise

Exercise, food, and your attitude are important to improve your sex life. Consider the following exercises, which can help you improve your sexual activity and performance. Start with these exercises only when you feel comfortable. Usually this will be around six weeks after you have had surgery.

Brisk Walking

People who are involved in aerobic exercise have a lower risk of developing problems with erections. Brisk walking helps to improve blood flow to the organs in your pelvis and therefore improves sexual function and performance. Do start to increase your speed gradually, as your body needs to recover after surgery.

Swimming

As soon as you feel comfortable, you can start visiting the swimming pool. Start with wading through the water and gradually get back to normal swimming. This is the best form of exercise, especially after weight-loss surgery, and for people with hip or knee problems.

Weight Lifting

Strength training exercises can help to improve your muscle mass and the muscles used in any sexual activity. Gradually increase the weight and intensity during any strength training exercises. Heavy weights, push-ups, and abdominal crunches should only be commenced after discussion with your doctor.

Kegels

Kegels help to improve the tone of your pubococcygeus muscles, which form part of your pelvic floor. This muscle helps to control ejaculation. Kegels are performed by contracting the muscle used to interrupt the flow of urine. Try it first in the bathroom. Thereafter, try doing it either in bed or sitting on the sofa. Contract and hold the muscle for ten seconds, relax, and gradually increase the repetitions.

Yoga

You can start doing yoga after you have recovered from weight-loss surgery. Yoga increases your stamina, flexibility, and the strength of your pelvic muscles. This can also help with sexual functioning.

Chapter 12
Pre-conception and Pregnancy after Bariatric Surgery

Pregnancy after bariatric surgery is becoming increasingly common. Many women of childbearing age have bariatric surgery to help improve their fertility or eligibility for in-vitro fertilisation (IVF) treatment, as they have often been unable to conceive naturally due to their obesity.

If you have had bariatric surgery, you will probably have experienced significant weight loss in the first year. Your body will be undergoing rapid changes. Your mind will be taking time to adjust to your new body. You will also need nutritional supplements to prevent vitamin and mineral deficiencies. Getting pregnant during this stage may not be safe for you and your baby, and for weight loss. It is therefore recommended that pregnancy should be delayed for at least 12-18 months after bariatric surgery.

After bariatric surgery, many women often ask about the potential health risks to the baby and themselves. However, increasing evidence suggests that the risks of having a baby after bariatric surgery are less when compared to the risks associated with being significantly overweight and pregnant.

Pregnancy after Bariatric Surgery

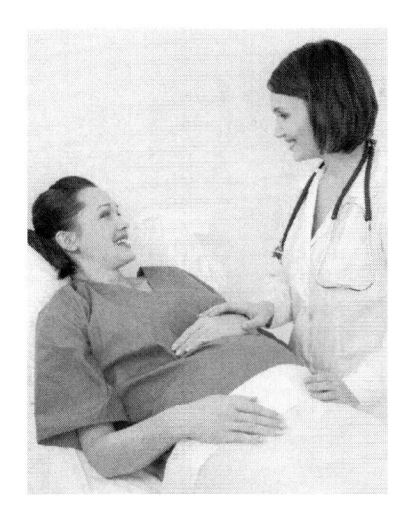

Pregnancy is not recommended for at least 12-18 months after bariatric surgery. This is because your body needs time to adjust to the weight loss and ensure that your diet is varied and as nutritious as possible to meet the needs of you and your baby. By waiting for at least 12-18 months after bariatric surgery to have a baby, you will also have a significant reduction in the health risks associated with obesity and pregnancy.

If you are planning a pregnancy, or are pregnant following bariatric surgery, you should inform your doctor and also your bariatric centre and dietitian. You should advise your doctor and midwife which bariatric surgery procedure that you have had. This will enable you to access the maternity services that you need and be monitored appropriately. It is also important to ensure that you have close monitoring by a dietitian to ensure your diet is as nutritious as possible and that you have regular micronutrient blood and weight monitoring.

Contraception

During the first 12 -18 months after bariatric surgery, it is recommended that contraceptive precautions are taken. The effectiveness of the contraceptive pill may be reduced after a malabsorptive procedure such as a gastric bypass or BPD+/-DS. You should seek medical advice upon the most appropriate contraception for you. Other types of contraception such as the implant (Implanon), coil, diaphragm, and condoms are not affected by surgery and are therefore safe to use.

Weight Gain during Pregnancy

Weight gain is expected during pregnancy, even after bariatric surgery. As with all pregnancies, how much you gain is individual to you. Some women can struggle to come to terms with weight gain during pregnancy when they have had a bariatric procedure to lose weight.

If you have concerns about your weight, you should consult your doctor or dietitian for support and advice. Try not to weigh yourself each day or every week as this can often create negative thoughts around your weight and you may forget about the positive aspects of having a baby and following a healthy lifestyle.

You should expect to have steady weight gain during pregnancy but avoid a significant amount of rapid weight gain as this may increase the health risks to you and your baby. If you eat a healthy diet and follow the dietary advice from your dietitian you should have steady weight gain. After you have had your baby, you should be able to lose any weight gained if you go back to the diet and physical activity levels that you had before pregnancy.

Monitoring during Pregnancy

Women who become pregnant after bariatric surgery are likely to be offered more frequent monitoring by their midwife and doctor. This monitoring may include more regular blood tests and foetal growth scans. You should have your micronutrient bloods checked during your pregnancy to prevent or correct any nutritional deficiencies.

What monitoring you have, and how often, will vary from person to person and the area in which you live. Most maternity units will provide you with your own hand held maternity notes. You should take these to all your maternity appointments to ensure that everyone that you see is able to record your pregnancy progress and share information.

Gestational Diabetes and Glucose Tolerance Tests

Gestational diabetes can occur after bariatric surgery. It is more common in people who have a BMI over 30kg/m². However it is still important to remember that your risk of developing gestational diabetes after bariatric surgery will be reduced because of the weight loss that you have had.

Depending upon your BMI and past medical history, you may be asked by your doctor to have a glucose tolerance test for gestational diabetes. This usually involves drinking a high-sugar containing drink over a specific period of time and having your blood glucose levels checked at timed intervals.

If you have had a gastric bypass or BPD +/-DS you may experience dumping syndrome with high sugar containing foods. If you know you experience dumping syndrome it is advisable that you discuss alternative methods of monitoring your blood glucose levels with your midwife and doctor.

Vitamin and Mineral Supplementation: Pre-conception and During Pregnancy

As with all pregnancies, it is not advisable to take a vitamin and mineral supplement that contains vitamin A, unless it is from a beta-carotene source. You should take a pre-conception or pregnancy specific multi-vitamin and mineral supplement, together with folic acid. Some doctors and dietitians may recommend a higher folic acid dose of 5mg.

You should consult your doctor or dietitian to determine what other nutritional supplements you may need. If you have been previously advised to have routine vitamin B12 injections following a gastric bypass, sleeve gastrectomy or DS+/-BPD, then you should continue with these.

You should contact your dietitian or doctor as soon as possible to find out what nutritional supplementation you will need to take to meet you and your baby's nutritional needs.

During Pregnancy

You should have your vitamin and mineral blood levels checked regularly during your pregnancy. Some bariatric centres recommend that you should have monthly blood checks. This will identify if you require any extra nutritional supplements to support you and your baby. If you are unsure which nutritional supplements you may need and what dose to take consult your doctor, dietitian or midwife.

Morning Sickness, Nausea and Vomiting During Pregnancy

Morning sickness is a common occurrence during any pregnancy whether you have had bariatric surgery or not. It is more common in the first 12-14 weeks of pregnancy; after then symptoms of nausea and vomiting generally reduce and stop.

If your dietary and fluid intake has become more limited because of nausea and vomiting related to your pregnancy you should consult your doctor, midwife or dietitian for advice.

Some women who suffer from pregnancy related nausea and vomiting may find eating little and often easier to tolerate. By eating little and often it may help to work out which foods reduce the symptoms of nausea and vomiting.

If you have pregnancy related nausea and vomiting try not to worry too much about eating a healthy, balanced diet at this stage. The main priority is to prevent becoming dehydrated. Some women find sipping on iced water, diluted fruit cordial, iced lollies, meal replacement drinks, soups and still diet drinks easier to manage.

If you feel that you are not drinking enough or have concerns about how limited your dietary intake is you should consult with your doctor or midwife.

Healthy Eating during Pregnancy

It is important to try to follow the pregnancy and healthy eating advice that your dietitian, doctor, or midwife recommend. However, after bariatric surgery, it can be often difficult to meet all of these recommendations due to the restriction on portion sizes and types of foods that are tolerated easier than others. It is advisable to try to follow the advice given, based upon what you feel is appropriate to the amount and types of foods you could eat before you became pregnant.

If you are finding that your diet is more limited than what it was like before your pregnancy you should try eating little and often, rather than rely on three tea-plate-sized meals per day. By eating four to six smaller meals per day, you should be able to have a better quality and varied diet. Some people use nutritious liquids or milk as one or two of their small meals per day as a way of combining fluid and nutrients in one.

After bariatric surgery, most pregnant women report that they often feel fuller quicker as their pregnancy progresses and the baby becomes bigger. Therefore many find eating smaller more frequent meals helps with this.

There is no special diet that you need to follow if you are planning a pregnancy or are pregnant. You should aim to eat a varied, healthy nutritious diet, which contains different foods every day. This should be the same as your bariatric surgery diet if you are at least 12-18 months after surgery.

You should aim to eat a combination of protein rich foods, such as meat, fish, peas, beans and lentils, eggs and dairy foods, together with starchy carbohydrates from pasta, rice, cereals and bread type products and fruit and vegetables.

You should avoid missing meals or going for long periods of time without having anything to eat or drink as this will not only reduce your energy levels but also limit how much nutrition you and your baby receive, particularly when your portion sizes are already limited after bariatric surgery. You will still need to avoid high fat and sugar containing foods, as you were advised before pregnancy.

Food Cravings

Like most other pregnant women, women who become pregnant after bariatric surgery can report food cravings. These food cravings can vary from person to person. It is important that you still include a variety of other nutritious foods and fluids to ensure you and your baby receive the nutrition that you need. Food cravings during pregnancy tend to last for short periods of time, before either moving onto another food or stopping altogether. If you have any concerns about your food cravings consult your midwife, doctor or dietitian for advice.

Breastfeeding

The benefits of breastfeeding are widely documented. These benefits include improved immunity to infections for your baby, suitable nutrition that is better absorbed compared to formula milk and a reduced risk of your baby becoming obese or developing type 2 diabetes in later life. Breastfeeding can use approximately 500kcals/day, which can also help with weight loss after pregnancy.

Most doctors and midwives will recommend that you breastfeed your baby, whether you have had bariatric surgery or not. However this advice will vary on an individual basis.

The nutritional adequacy of breast milk in women following bariatric surgery is unknown. If you are planning to breastfeed your baby or if you are unsure whether to breastfeed or use infant formula, you should discuss this with your doctor and or midwife/dietitian before delivery.

You should check whether you continue with any nutritional supplementation that you have been taking during your pregnancy.

Most bariatric centres will advise you about appropriate nutritional supplementation and have your vitamin and mineral blood levels re-checked and monitored.

Constipation during Pregnancy

Constipation is common during any pregnancy irrespective of whether or not you have bariatric surgery. It is important to ensure that you drink at least two litres of fluid per day. If you do not drink enough fluid each day this can be the main cause of constipation. You should also ensure that you have good sources of fibre in your diet. Sources of fibre include peas, beans and lentils, fruit and vegetables and wholegrain cereals.

If you feel that you have a good amount of fluid and fibre in your diet, but still have symptoms of constipation you should consult with your doctor or midwife about taking medication.

Gastric Band Adjustments during Pregnancy

Gastric band adjustment advice during pregnancy can vary between bariatric centres. Some bariatric centres will advise all pregnant women with a gastric band to have their band emptied during pregnancy, to enable them to choose a good quality, nutritious diet. However, other centres may not loosen the band unless there are problems of frequent vomiting and/or an overly restrictive gastric band diet, which is then not suitable to meet you and your baby's nutritional needs. Some bariatric units will recommend that you keep some fluid in your gastric band to help control large amounts of weight gain during pregnancy, which increases the health risks associated with the weight gain to you and your baby. You should still be able to manage a varied diet and tea plate sized portions.

If you do not have your band emptied during pregnancy, it can sometimes become more difficult to determine whether frequent vomiting and an overly restrictive diet is related to the pregnancy or the gastric band itself. There have been some reports of an increased risk of gastric band slippage during pregnancy. Remember you will not be able to have a radiological (x-ray) band adjustment during pregnancy to check the band position.

As soon as you know that you are pregnant you should consult your bariatric centre for advice about what to do about your gastric band restriction and whether it is appropriate to empty or adjust the gastric band.

Chapter 13
Weight Regain after Bariatric Surgery

Weight regain can happen for some people after bariatric surgery. It is more likely to occur two to five years after having bariatric surgery.

Usually there is nothing wrong with the bariatric surgery. Rather, it is likely that as time has gone by, it can be easy to slip back into old eating habits, such as snacking and/or increasing portion sizes or reducing your physical activity levels. The main reasons or triggers for weight regain are:

- Family, friend, work problems or stresses which have led to emotional/comfort eating.
- Set unrealistic expectations and goals on what the weight loss would achieve.
- Expected greater weight loss and/or health benefits associated with the weight loss.
- Expected that the weight loss would change your home/work/family circumstances.
- Did not change food choices or eating habits.
- Did not increase physical activity levels.
- Did not establish a regular meal pattern and continued to miss meals or eat late at night.
- Increased alcohol intake.

This chapter will help you consider the changes that you need to make to reduce your energy intake and increase your physical activity levels to get back on track with your weight loss or make you aware of the pitfalls that some people fall into after bariatric surgery, to help you prevent falling into these yourself.

You may have stretched your stomach/gastric pouch by not following the dietary advice and rules provided by your dietitian and bariatric centre.

As you can see from the diagram below, even after bariatric surgery if more calories are eaten than are used by your body, your weight will begin to increase. Excess calories eaten which are not used will be stored as fat.

Energy In vs. Energy Out: How the Body Maintains Weight

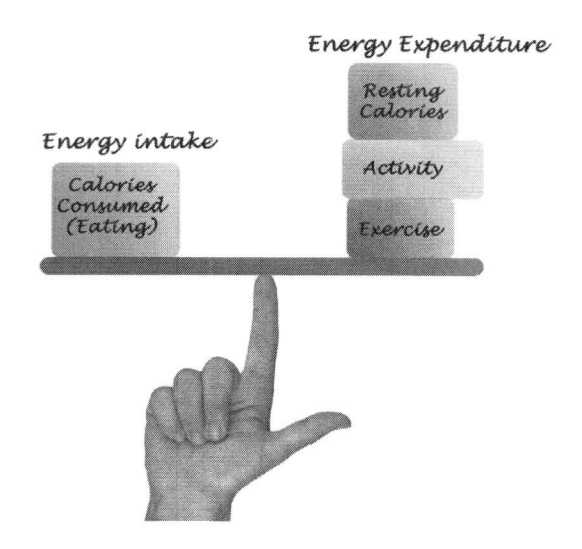

Energy Expenditure
- Resting Calories
- Activity
- Exercise

Energy intake
- Calories Consumed (Eating)

Weight

It is important to address weight regain as soon as possible in order to prevent any further weight regain and feel comfortable with your overall progress. Try not to go back to trying 'quick fix' diets that you may have tried in the past in an attempt to lose weight. This will not provide a long-term solution to your weight gain. You should seek advice from your dietitian and bariatric centre to get back on track.

Psychological Impact of Weight Regain

Re-gaining weight after bariatric surgery can have a significant psychological and emotional impact on a person. He/she can feel depressed, anxious, and frustrated. They can also feel quite helpless and ashamed. In such circumstances, people tend to think badly about themselves, as if they are a failure and that they have let others down.

It is important to remember that such feelings and thoughts tend to lead people to eat more, not less. Such 'bad' feelings and thoughts can also prevent people seeking the help and support they need.

If you ignore your weight regain in the early stages, you may find that it becomes much more difficult to get control back of your eating and weight.

What to Do about Weight Regain

- Don't panic
- Do not ignore it
- Do seek help, including from the bariatric surgery service or a psychologist
- Speak to supportive friends and family
- Focus on the positive aspects of the weight loss you have achieved overall

There are a number of things that you can do to help control your weight in the longer term.

Recognising That You Feel Full

The most common sign of feeling full is experiencing discomfort, nausea or pain around your breastbone area. This is a signal to stop eating. Try to stop eating just before you get to this point. It can take sometime getting used to this. If you are having trouble with recognising the feeling of fullness, try to use some portion guidelines to help you get used to how much food will be enough for your stomach/gastric pouch.

Use a Tea Plate to Control Your Portion Sizes

As a guideline, use a small tea plate/side plate (16cm diameter). Don't present your food on a larger plate than this, as a larger plate will encourage you to eat more. Some people before bariatric surgery have always had to eat everything off their plate, despite feeling full. Using a tea plate will help you self-monitor your portion sizes, rather than visually estimating portion sizes on a larger plate.

Don't Go Back to Meals after Feeling Full or Vomiting

Some people go back to meals after feeling full or vomiting. If you have anything left on your plate, either save it for another meal or throw it away, so the temptation to go back and eat the rest of the food isn't there.

It should take you approximately 15-20 minutes to eat a solid textured tea-plate sized meal. If you keep stopping and going back to your meals, you are tricking the bariatric surgery operation, so that you feel less dietary restriction. This will therefore allow you to eat more food and calories and lead to less than expected weight loss and weight gain.

Going back to meals soon after feeling full may also stretch your stomach/gastric pouch.

Eat More Solid Textured Foods

Some people tend to choose softer, melt in the mouth foods as these are easier to tolerate and can cause a less uncomfortable feeling when eaten. Soft foods will not help make you feel full and are likely to be higher in calories. Solid textured foods help reduce your portion size eaten and make you feel fuller for longer, reducing your appetite.

Soft, Melt in the Mouth Foods

Weight regain is often caused by eating (grazing) on soft, melt in the mouth foods more often and usually in place of sitting down and eating a planned meal. Snack type foods are those that tend to be high in fat and/or energy (crisps, chocolate, ice cream, biscuits and sweets) all of which should be eaten least often or rarely.

These foods glide through the pouch/stomach very easily and don't make you feel full or reduce your appetite.

Don't Take Food and Fluid Together

It is not advisable to take food and fluid together, even if you are able to do this. Drinks or sauces (gravy, mayonnaise, salad dressings etc.) help 'wash' more food through the stomach/gastric pouch which increases the calories eaten but also it can stretch your pouch and not reduce your appetite. Stretching your gastric pouch/stomach will increase your portion sizes and calorie content of your diet, leading to weight gain.

Increasing Physical Activity Levels

Physical activity is an important part of your lifestyle change. People who build exercise into their lifestyle after bariatric surgery tend to have better overall weight loss and keep the weight off long term.

As you lose weight you will become more mobile and you will be able to do things more easily. It is important to continue to build on these activities and find new activities that you enjoy as time goes on. Choose an activity that you can fit into your lifestyle that you can maintain in the longer-term.

Getting Back on Track with Your Diet

There are a number of ways to get back on track to help control your appetite, dietary intake and reduce your weight. With all the bariatric surgery procedures, you should eat up to three, tea-plate sized portions of solid, textured foods.

The ways to increase the texture of your diet, to help reduce the portion size and make you feel fuller for longer are:

- Eat the right way round your tea plate. Eat the most textured part of your meal first rather than leave it until last. Eat the meat of a roast dinner first, then eat the vegetables and potato last and use less gravy; you should find that you feel full quicker and for longer.
- Choose more foods off the caution list. These include meat, bread, pasta, rice, salad, fibrous fruit, and vegetables.
- Add less sauce, gravy or salad dressings to foods, as liquid will 'wash' food through the gastric pouch/stomach and enable you to tolerate more food and calories, and not reduce your appetite for long enough.
- Do not overcook vegetables, mash them up, or add extra gravy.
- If having a jacket potato or crackers/crisp breads, add some salad to them to increase the texture to help you feel full quicker and for longer.
- If you are tempted to snack, choose fruit or cereal bars with dried fruit/oats or raw vegetables such as carrot, celery, cucumber, peppers.
- If having soups, choose ones with chunky vegetables and pasta/rice or meat. Avoid smooth, thin soups as this will glide through the gastric pouch or stomach and not make you feel full.

- If you are having yogurt or breakfast cereal, add fruit to increase the texture to help you make you feel full quicker and for longer.

- Drink low calorie liquids 30 minutes before and after meals. If you are tempted to snack, try having a low calorie drink or water instead.

Where Can I Get Support for Weight Regain after Weight-Loss Surgery?

There are a number of places you can go for support if you experience weight regain. These include:

- The bariatric dietitian
- Your family doctor (who can refer you back to the bariatric team if necessary)
- Weight management support groups (either from the hospital or in your local community)
- **simply***bariatrics*.com

Chapter 14
Your Relationship with Food

Preface

As already outlined in this book, obesity is complex and effective treatments vary between individuals. Simply having bariatric surgery cannot guarantee weight loss and lifelong maintenance, unless you are willing to change your lifestyle.

In many cases, where people are seeking treatment, including surgery, for obesity, a clinical psychologist or therapist can help support and make the necessary lifestyle changes. By understanding what your relationship to food is, and how to change it, any weight loss operation is likely to be more successful.

*This chapter has been written by **Dr Adam Saradjian,** who is a senior clinical psychologist specialising in obesity management. He presents an overview of how and why we eat, how we can manage our relationship with food, and provides some useful tools to help you with your weight loss journey.*

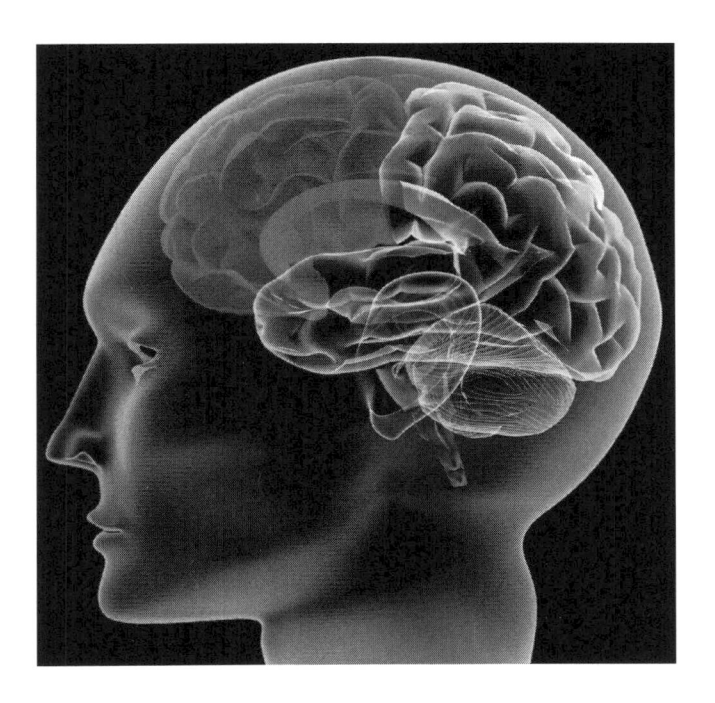

Introduction

Let's make it clear from the very start; nobody **only** eats or drinks when they are hungry or thirsty.

Everyone eats and drinks to help change how they feel.

In fact, *everything* we do is intended to either get (or keep) a feeling that we *want*, or change a feeling that we *don't* want. That is part of being human. So, if we get pleasure from something, of course we want more of it.

Humans are built to find eating pleasurable and satisfying, because if they didn't, they wouldn't eat, and if they didn't eat, the human race would die. Indeed, with the increasing availability of different foods from across the world, we have got better at combining and preparing food to make it taste even more delicious.

Food and drink is much more readily available these days and we gain great pleasure from shopping for food, not just from cooking or eating it.

The term **'comfort eating'** is commonly used to mean "turning to food" to make us feel better when we are down. Although true, this can also be an over-simplistic way of thinking about it. For example, whatever we are eating and drinking can help us switch our attention from other things we have on our mind, that perhaps feel stressful, messy, and difficult to sort out.

Focusing our attention and senses on food distracts us from these problems, and (at least in the short-term) gives us a sense of relief from our stresses. This feeling becomes associated with *eating* as if in some way the food has actually contributed to solving problems.

Eating food can be a highly social activity throughout our lives: whether it is as an infant being fed by his mother or child having a birthday cake and meal out to celebrate her birthday. Alternatively, food may have 'been there' for us when others haven't. In summary, food has many associations and serves many different 'functions' or needs.

Given the fact that you are reading this, food is likely to have played an important role throughout your life in some way or another.

This chapter is aimed at helping you better understand your personal relationship with food. Only once you understand something can you really begin to change how you behave, and maintain this change.

This chapter also contains a specially designed food diary to help you develop your understanding, and a personal action plan to help you change your relationship with food and learn to meet your needs more often through ways other than eating/drinking.

Understanding How Things Will Change Following Weight-Loss Surgery.

It is important to understand how life and relationships may change following weight-loss surgery. Many people think that surgery will automatically make our lives better and happier, and that we will no longer desire as much food.

Surgery *will* change *how* much you are able to eat, and your relationship with food to some degree, but it **does not** mean that you won't be drawn to food in the same way that you have been in the past. As already highlighted, this is because we do not *only* eat when we are hungry and therefore this will not necessarily change after weight-loss surgery.

When food has played an important part in our lives, the inability to eat in the same way that we did before surgery is likely to feel like a significant loss. Food may have been a main source of pleasure, comfort, or way of socialising with others. After surgery, if we can no longer experience these "pleasures" as much with food, what then?

Weight-loss surgery is an effective 'tool' to help achieve weight loss and improve health. The diary and the personal action plan contained in this chapter can help you with your weight-loss surgery journey. It can also help you to develop a more balanced and satisfying life.

Relationship with Food

People often say that they have a love-hate relationship with food. They are talking about how much they *feel* like they need food, but also that they suffer a number of 'bad' or unintended consequences from eating 'too much'.

The good tends to be experienced in the short-term, and the bad tends to be experienced in the long-term. The lack of control and feelings of dependency to meet your needs also leads to feeling like you 'hate' food as well as 'love' it.

People need food and drink to live, so unlike other things we turn to for comfort (like drinking alcohol or smoking cigarettes), nobody can stop eating altogether. This means that since it is not possible to remove food entirely from life, we must learn to become 'friends' with food. To develop a friendship with food, we must better understand our relationship with food, and thus better understand ourselves.

The Relationship with Food Diary

Many people who are trying to lose weight will have filled in (or at least been asked to fill in) food diaries, so why do another one? The diary included in this chapter is a psychologically-based one, aimed at helping you to understand *why* you tend to eat more, rather than just about *how much*. It helps you consider what role food plays in meeting our human needs for pleasure, satisfaction, comfort and social connection.

It is well recognised by psychologists that 'regulation', or the ability to control something, involves monitoring and then modifying accordingly. Writing things in a diary is a helpful way of monitoring because it is hard to keep track of everything without recording it.

Recording helps us recognise and examine patterns, so we can have more insight into what we are doing. We can then look at how to change things to help us to meet our goals.

The diary is intended for use in an initial period of two weeks to one month; however, you may also use the diary if you ever feel like you are struggling to meet your goals.

Although not indicated in the diary, remember that the way in which you eat strongly influences what and how much you eat. If you eat too quickly and do not really pay attention to the taste and texture of food, you may eat more. In addition, eating quickly does not give enough time for your brain to tell you that it is 'full' and it may also make you vomit.

However, if you snack and eat small amounts of food slowly, you are also likely to eat more because your stomach will have less chance to feel 'full'. Eating small amounts often can be known as 'nibbling' or 'grazing'. It is therefore important that you follow the advised dietary rules, as you may regain weight in the longer term if you eat like this.

Guidance on Completing the Diary

Below is some guidance on filling in the different sections of the diary. There is also an example (see figure 1), which gives you an idea of what the diary looks like.

Try to complete the diary whenever you eat or drink, so you remember everything that you ate and when. If you leave the diary until the end of the day or the next day to complete, it may not be an accurate reflection of your day. If your diary is inaccurate or incomplete it may not work as intended and it will not support you.

Figure 1. Relationship with Food Diary

Relationship with Food Diary

Day/Date/Time	Situation Inc. if mealtime	Emotion/Feelings	Automatic Thoughts	Food/Drink Consumed	Consequent Emotions/Feelings	Consequent Automatic Thoughts/Judgements

Your own diary may look similar or very different from the example, however as long as the diary helps you to understand your patterns of eating/drinking then it is working for you.

It is not a diary to repeatedly complete, but neither is it intended to be a diary that you record and never develop a plan from.

Situation: This means asking yourself "where are you and what are you doing"? For example, you may be at home watching television; you may have just got off the phone to someone who has talked to you about their problems; you may have just got back from work; you may be out shopping and stop at a café; or it could be a mealtime either at home or out. It is also helpful here to include if you are on your own or with others, and if so, who.

Emotion/Feelings: What are you feeling now? You may be feeling stressed, tired, worried, anxious, fed-up, ashamed, guilty, angry, bored, numb, happy, excited or hungry. Sometimes you may not know what you are feeling at the time. In this case record it, and then maybe look back later and try to think about what you were feeling. If this is a common occurrence, this in itself may be contributing to your problems—you don't **know** what you are feeling.

Automatic Thoughts: In this situation, with these feelings, what pops into your head now? What are you thinking? What are you feeling?

For example, are you worried or happy about something? What are you thinking as you are about to eat/drink? It may be simply that "I'm hungry, I need something to eat". Or it could be that there is a lot swirling around in your head and it seems hard to capture, but this is a skill that can be learnt with practice and may be helpful.

Food/Drink Consumed: What and how much have you eaten or drunk? Here you can be as detailed or not as you like. You may want to record calories, but perhaps it is easier just to record this information more roughly, unless specifically guided to by a dietitian.

Consequent Emotions/Feelings: Having finished eating/drinking, how are you feeling? It may be the same as those noted above, or could it include others about how you are feeling. Has eating or drinking made you feel disappointed, angry, guilty, fed-up, down, anxious, pleased, satisfied, or proud? You may notice that you feel a certain way initially and then something else shortly afterwards. You may also want to include any change in emotion, i.e., do you feel 'better' or 'worse' than you did before eating? Also notice if the feeling you have now is what you intended or expected to feel before eating or not.

Consequent Automatic Thoughts/Judgements: Now that you have finished eating or drinking, with this feeling, what pops into your head? What are you thinking? What are you, for example, angry or pleased about? It is also important here to include any 'judgements' you may be making about yourself. How do you think or feel about yourself now?

Learning From Your Diary

You may notice some patterns keep recurring as you fill in the diary. You may notice others when you look back at a day, a week, or even longer. You may realise that there are certain times of day you tend to 'overeat'. For many it is in the evening that we snack. It may also be that during the week, things are not 'too bad' but then 'it all becomes out of control' at the weekend. There may be particular places or situations that you tend to eat more. For some it could be at home, for others when out, or even in your car. There may be some common moods with feelings and thoughts that lead you to eating more. Eating may change this mood and how you see yourself, but perhaps not in the way that you intended beforehand.

Learning to Meet Your Needs More Appropriately

Once you have completed the food diary, you will hopefully have a better understanding and record of your relationship with food and your patterns of eating and drinking. Now you need to understand what you need to do to change things. This involves learning to meet your needs in other ways, rather than relying too much on food and drink to meet these needs.

It is important to develop a plan to help minimise overeating and learn to respond differently, with a greater sense of choice and control than before. This plan would be developed from the understanding that you have gained from the diary.

It is important to realise that nobody can have all their needs met all of the time. However, if you become more aware of your needs, you can learn to meet them more often than you have been in other ways than with food and drink.

Below is some guidance on developing your own personal action plan to meet your needs more appropriately. You may initially find this plan difficult to work through on your own and so if you can, it would be useful to get the advice and help of any trusted and supportive friends and family.

Trigger to Overeat, Feeling—Need: There are likely to be particular times, situations, feelings or moods that 'trigger' you to overeat, not thinking or caring about what or how much you are eating. You will hopefully have a good understanding of these having used the 'relationship with food diary'.

Figure 2. Example of a completed Relationship with Food Diary

Day/Date/Time	Situation Inc. if mealtime	Emotion/Feelings	Automatic Thoughts	Food/Drink Consumed	Consequent Emotions/Feelings	Consequent Automatic Thoughts/Judgements
2.30pm	Snack On bus home	Stressed Fed up	I need some chocolate now	Chocolate Diet coke	More relaxed at first, then annoyed at self	What's the point?
5.00pm	Tea at home	Alright	Right I need to be 'good' now	Weight Watchers ready made lasagne No sugar squash drink	Alright, maybe some disappointment	That wasn't very nice, what else can I have, but no I shouldn't have anything else
Evening	Snack at home watching TV	Tired Bored Lonely Sad	I need something, forget the diet	x4 bags of crisps x4 choc chip biscuits x 2 teas	Disappointed and annoyed at myself	I'm useless I'll be 'good' tomorrow

List these known 'triggers' in the first column. It is important that you recognise the need associated with the trigger situation or feeling. For example, if you are highly stressed, the associated "need" is to 'unwind' or relax; if you are bored or fed up you may "need" pleasure, stimulation or something 'to do'; if you are anxious, you may "need" reassurance or calming.

Warning Signs & Situations Associated with Overeating: In the 'heat of the moment' it can be difficult to be aware of the warning signs and situations. Therefore, to help you in such times, it is important to have cues to look out for. It is also helpful to separate these into internal and external warning signs. *'Internal'* refers more to what and where you feel things in your body. Examples may include feeling restless or 'on edge', having fidgety hands or feet, feeling empty inside, feeling like you've got 'butterflies in your stomach'. Internal also includes common thoughts you may have that are associated with overeating such as "I'm a failure", "I don't deserve to be happy", "and I'll be 'good' tomorrow". *'External'* refers more to the situations that give rise to the trigger feelings such as being home alone; having had an argument with someone, feeling worthless or spending lots of time listening to other people's problems.

Physical and Psychological Consequences of Meeting Need with Food: It is important to be clear in your mind what would be the 1) physical and the 2) psychological consequences if you were to meet the "need" with food. These should be separated into the short term and the longer term.

Alternatives to Overeating to Meet the Identified Need or Response to Feeling: This is about developing a 'menu' of different choices to meet your needs more appropriately. It is very important that you have a variety of different options because different situations require different things. For example, if you like to have a bath to help you relax, what if you weren't at home and needed to relax? Some things to consider when developing your menu are:

- Can you do this at home or outside?
- Can you do this on your own or with others?
- Do you need some equipment (like a television) for this activity?
- Is this something you can do already, or is it something you want to learn?

Whatever they are, they need to be important to you.

Implementing the Plan

It can often be hard to put plans into action, so you will need to consider this carefully and work out how best to start your plan. Changing long-standing automatic behaviours can be difficult and takes time. It can be helpful to make one or two changes at a time and really focus your efforts on establishing these before moving onto others. Whilst it is natural to feel disheartened about a lapse of falling into old habits, try not to dwell on this and think of yourself as a failure. Notice what has happened, try to learn from it, and refocus your efforts.

The plan needs to be somewhere easy to access, especially at first. It is also vital to share the plan with others close to you, so they can help you put it into action.

Conclusion

This chapter has provided some practical information, advice, and tools, which can help you achieve and maintain a healthier weight, and a better quality of life. On-going support and guidance from those around you is important to achieve positive results and meet your goals. Self-help tools such as the relationship with food diary can help support you to be more aware of the factors affecting your food choices and develop a realistic individualised plan to manage your triggers to eating and drinking.

Some people may need psychological help and support after weight-loss surgery. You may want to discuss this with your doctor or weight-loss surgery team. If you want to pursue psychological therapy, it is recommended that you should ensure that the therapist is appropriately registered and accredited with a nationally recognised professional body.

Chapter 15
Food Groups: Protein, Fat, and Carbs

Protein, fat, and carbohydrate are the three main food groups. All three food groups are important to include in the diet after bariatric surgery. How much or little of these food groups that is needed in the diet depends upon individual dietary and health needs and the bariatric procedure done.

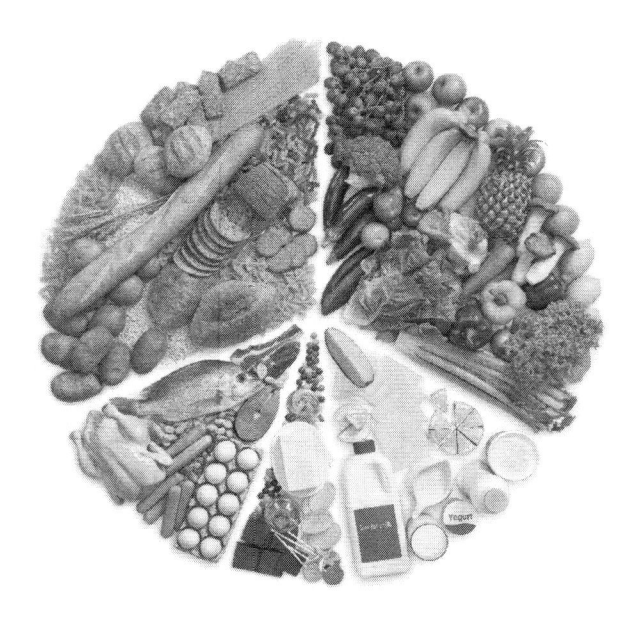

There may be some differences in the food group proportions depending upon your government's dietary guidelines and individual health needs.

Protein

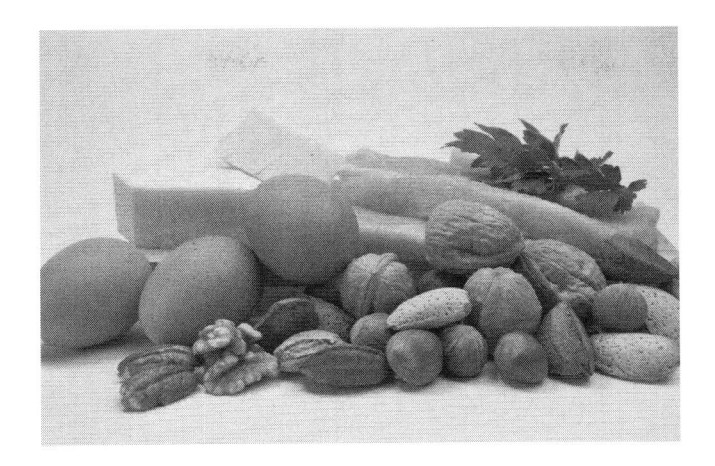

Protein is made of amino acids; these are essential or non-essential amino acids. Non-essential amino acids are made by your body and essential amino acids have to be obtained from your diet.

Protein is needed for many bodily functions including:

- Muscle and tissue repair (including heart and lungs)
- Healthy hair, skin and nails
- Healthy immune system
- Minimise muscle mass reduction during weight loss

Where is protein found?

Protein is found in animal products, such as meat, milk, cheese, eggs, and fish; and as plant protein in peas, beans, and lentils. Animal protein is a better source of protein for your body than plant protein;

however, animal proteins can be higher in fat while plant proteins are low in fat, high in fibre, and contain vitamins and minerals.

How much protein should you eat per day?

The amount of protein that you are advised to aim for per day will vary depending upon what bariatric procedure you have had and what stage of the diet you are following after your operation. Generally, as a guide, the advice based upon current recommendations is to aim for 60-70g of protein per day. If you have had a BPD+/- DS the advice is to aim for between 80-90g of protein per day.

What foods are high in protein?

In the early stages after bariatric surgery, most people find that dairy-based (milk, eggs, cheese and yogurt) and plant-based protein foods easier to manage. This is because these protein sources tend to be soft or liquid as in milk-based products or peas, beans, and lentils that can be cooked so they are very soft or pureed.

Meat can be one of the most difficult foods to tolerate after bariatric surgery, even in the longer term. Some people can manage minced or stewed meat or use soya protein meat alternative products.

It is important to try and include protein at meal times, particularly in the early stages after surgery, whilst you recover. Protein will help your wounds heal and the swelling from your surgery reduce quicker.

Protein Content of Some Foods

The amount and texture of protein you can tolerate in your diet will vary depending upon what bariatric surgery operation you have had and how long ago you had your surgery.

Below is a list of some protein rich foods:

- One portion of hard cheese (50g, 2oz, (1/4 cup): 12g protein.
- One medium egg: 6g protein.
- 568mls (1 pint) of milk: 18g protein.
- 100g, 4oz (1/2 cup) yogurt: 10g protein
- One tablespoon of boiled red lentils (40g): 3g protein.
- One portion of tofu (125g): 15g protein.
- 50g, 2oz (1/4 cup) lean minced beef: 7g protein.
- 50g, 20oz (1/4 cup) soya protein mince: 7g protein
- Half a chicken breast (65g): 20g protein.
- Small, poached, skinless fish fillet (75g): 18g protein.
- Half a can of tuna: 19g protein.

Carbohydrates

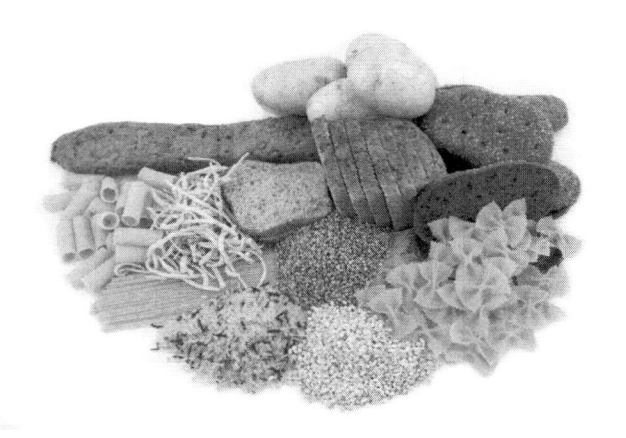

Carbohydrates can be split into two groups: complex carbohydrates (such as potato, bread, pasta, couscous and rice) and simple carbohydrates (such as table sugar, jam, sweets, desserts, and sugary drinks).

Complex carbohydrates are important part your diet to provide energy. Complex carbohydrates should be part of your meals. Once you have established your diet in the longer term, approximately one quarter of your tea plate should contain complex carbohydrates.

After bariatric surgery, you should avoid simple carbohydrates in food and fluids. Simple carbohydrates can cause dumping syndrome following a gastric bypass or DS+/-BPD. Simple carbohydrate food and fluids tend to contain very little (if any) nutrition. Artificial sweeteners (such as Splenda, Sweet and Low, and Canderel) can be used as an alternative to sugar, as they do not cause dumping syndrome or contain calories.

Fat

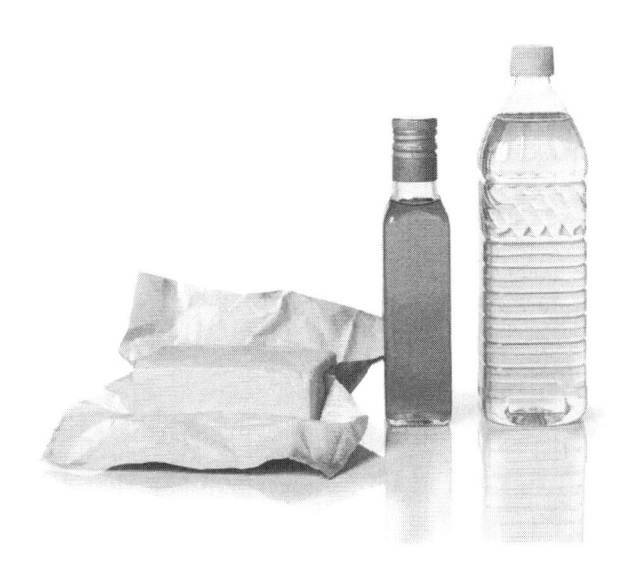

Fat is a concentrated source of energy (calories). Foods, which contain fat, should be eaten in small amounts, but should not be avoided.

Fats can be split into three main types. These are:

1. Saturated fats such as butter, cream and lard.
2. Polyunsaturated fats found in nut and seed oils
3. Monounsaturated fats such as olive, corn and sunflower oils

Some fats are better than others to include in your diet to benefit your health. These fats are mono and polyunsaturated fats. Fats provide important vitamins (A, D, E, K), which are needed by your body to be healthy. It is important to remember that all types of fats contain the same amount of calories per gram.

Some people can experience steatorrhoea (fatty diarrhoea) following some bariatric procedures, namely the DS +/_ BPD and gastric bypass. Steatorrhoea is caused by eating too much fat. If you eat a low fat diet with any of the bariatric procedures, you should lose weight and prevent steatorrhoea. A low fat diet should be 3g per 100g or 3 percent fat or less.

Chapter 16

Recipes

This section provides some recipe ideas, which may help ensure a good variety of food and food groups in the diet. For further recipe ideas and information visit **simply**bariatrics.com.

Stage One — Liquids Only

It is important to drink plenty of fluids. This can often be difficult in the early stages after surgery when patients are only able to take small sips of liquids. Use a straw or a sports cap flask or bottle to help control how much fluid is consumed at any one time. It is important to include nutritious fluids at meal times.

The following are examples of fluids that should be included in the diet:

Meal Replacement Drinks

Meal replacement drinks are ideal for most people after bariatric surgery as they are generally high in protein and contain vitamins, minerals, and fibre. Meal replacement drinks can be bought in most supermarkets, pharmacies or on the Internet. Try to choose meal replacement drinks that are low in sugar and calories.

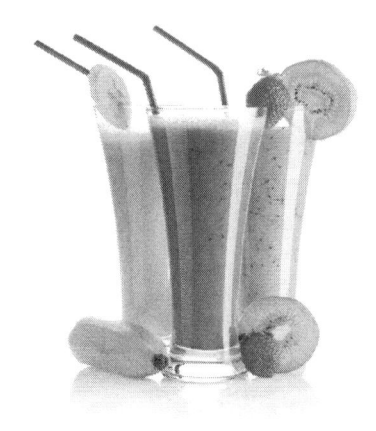

Smoothies

Smoothies can be a good way of providing vitamin, minerals, and fibre from fruit and vegetables during the liquid stage of the diet. Smoothies can either be bought or be made from different combinations of fruit and vegetables to suit individual taste. If fruit smoothies made at home rather than purchased, low fat/diet yoghurt or milk/powder can be added to increase protein.

Soups

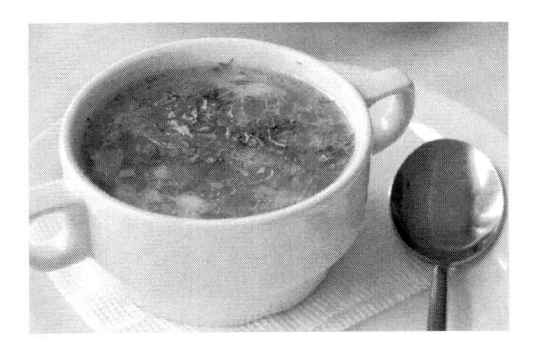

Soups are an ideal nutritious, versatile liquid. These can either be bought in the shops or made at home. Ensure that soups contain protein rich ingredients such as meat, fish, peas, beans, and lentils. Soups should be blended at this stage. If purchasing soups that have bits in, use a blender to make them smooth. Try not to sieve the soups instead of blending them, as this will remove some nutrition from the soup.

Stage One Recipes

Peach, Blueberry, Strawberry and Banana Smoothie

Ingredients

- 4 very ripe peaches or nectarines, sliced and skinned
- 50g (1/3 cup) frozen blueberries
- 50g, 2oz (1/3 cup) strawberries
- 1 large peeled and chopped banana,
- 6 tbsp low fat Greek yoghurt

Method

1. Place the peaches or nectarines into a juicer and extract the juice.
2. Pour the juice into a blender with the remaining ingredients and blend.
3. Serve.

Frozen Fruit Smoothie

Ingredients

- 1 large ripe banana, peeled and sliced
- 1 x 200ml glass frozen fruit (blueberries, raspberries, mango, redcurrants)
- 2 heaped tablespoons natural low fat yoghurt
- 15g (1 level tablespoon) rolled oats
- 1 x 200ml glass skimmed/semi skimmed milk

Method

1. Place the banana in the blender with the yoghurt and frozen fruit. Blend together.
2. Add the rolled oats and milk and blend again, until smooth. If you find the smoothie is too thick, add a little more milk to thin the smoothie.
3. Serve.

Vegetable and Blueberry Smoothie

Ingredients

- 9 oz (250g) frozen spinach, chopped
- 6 oz (170g) low fat/fat free blueberry yoghurt
- Half a ripe avocado, pitted and peeled
- 3/4 cup (180mls) cranberry-blueberry juice
- 1/2 cup (120g) frozen blueberries

Method

1. Microwave or steam the spinach as directed on the pack. Once cooked, rinse with cold water until cooled. Drain, squeezing out as much liquid as possible.
2. In a blender, place 1/4 cup of the cooked, squeezed spinach and all the remaining ingredients.
3. Blend until smooth.
4. Serve

For further recipe and meal ideas, please go to **simply***bariatrics*.com

Stage Two— Pureed

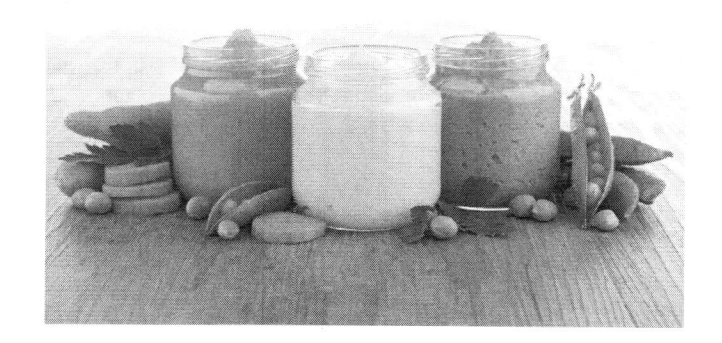

Stage two of the diet is pureed food. The pureed food should be a custard consistency. The portion sizes on this stage are approximately two to three tablespoons, initially. If meals are cooked and pureed using a blender, consider portioning meals into ice cube/small containers. This will allow convenient freezing, defrosting, and reheating of pureed food when needed, without wasting food. If reheated pureed food is a little thicker than desired, add extra gravy, white sauce, or milk to loosen up the pureed food a little and ensure the right consistency.

Most people prepare the pureed stage of the diet before having bariatric surgery. Every day meals, such as meat or fish, potato and vegetables, can be pureed ahead of time. Use herbs and spices to add extra flavour to the pureed food.

Stage Two Recipes

Chicken, Carrots and Potato Puree

Ingredients

- 1 small onion, peeled and chopped
- 350g/12oz (1.5 cups) carrots, peeled and sliced
- 250ml/8 fl oz chicken stock
- 125g/4oz (1/2 cup) 1 chicken breast, chopped into 1cm cubes
- 1 small potato, peeled and chopped into 1cm cubes
- low calorie vegetable/olive oil spray

Method

1. Heat a non-stick saucepan, add one spray of the low calorie oil and cook the onion until softened.
2. Add the sliced carrots and potato, pour over the chicken stock and bring to a boil.
3. Reduce the heat, then cover with a lid and cook for 10 minutes.
4. Add the chopped chicken breast and chopped carrots and continue to cook for 10 minutes.
5. Puree in a blender.
6. Serve.
7. Freeze the remainder as individual portions.

Lentil and Vegetable Puree

Ingredients

- 1 small onion, finely chopped
- 100g/4oz (1/2 cup) carrot, peeled and sliced
- 15g celery, chopped
- 50g/2oz (1/3 cup) split red lentils
- 200g/8oz (1 cup) potato, peeled and chopped into cubes
- 400ml, 14 fl oz vegetable or chicken stock
- Low calorie vegetable/olive oil spray

Method

1. Heat a non-stick saucepan, add one spray of the low calorie oil into the saucepan and cook the onion, carrot and celery until softened
2. Add the lentils and sweet potato, and then pour over the stock
3. Bring to the boil, turn down the heat and simmer covered with a lid for 20 minutes
4. Purée in a blender
5. Serve
6. Freeze the remainder as individual portions.

Stage Three—Soft, Mushy and Crispy

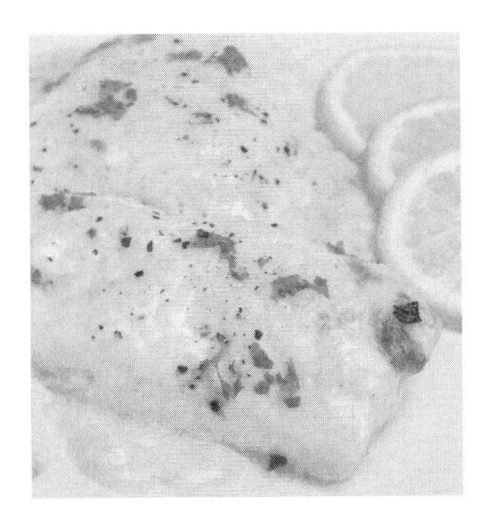

Stage three of the diet is soft, mushy and crispy. This stage the patient is ready to try more variety of textured foods with soft lumps in sauces and gravies. Crispy foods are foods that dissolve in water, such as crackers, crispbreads, breadsticks, and toast. These recipes can be used for family and friends without needing to change anything. The portion sizes of meals will vary at this stage depending upon the bariatric procedure and the time since the operation.

Stage Three Recipes

Cottage Pie

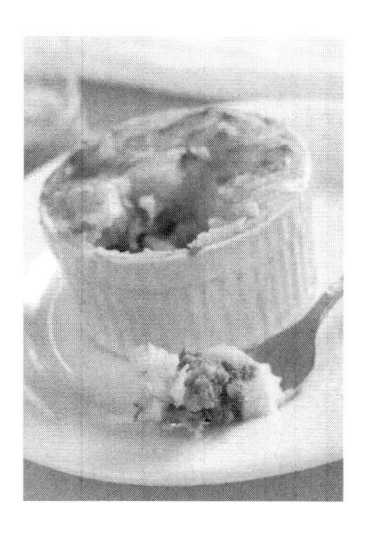

Ingredients

- 1 large onion, peeled and chopped finely
- 1 clove garlic, crushed
- 2 medium carrots, peeled and chopped finely
- 1 stick of celery, chopped finely
- 500g (2 1/2 cups) lean, minced beef
- 1 (400g, 2 cups) tin chopped tomatoes
- 2 tablespoons tomato purée
- 300ml (10 fl oz) beef stock
- 1 teaspoon dried mixed herbs
- low calorie vegetable/olive oil spray

- salt and freshly ground black pepper to taste

For the topping
- 1kg (4.5 cups), peeled and diced potato
- 4 tablespoons semi skimmed or skimmed milk

Method

1. Preheat the oven to 190 C / Gas mark 5.
2. Heat a large saucepan over a medium heat. Spray the vegetable, olive oil into the pan.
3. Add the onion, garlic, celery and carrot and cook over a medium heat until soft.
4. Add the mince and brown.
5. Add the tinned tomatoes, purée, beef stock, mixed herbs.
6. Season to taste with salt and pepper. Cover and simmer for 30 minutes.
7. Meanwhile, boil the potatoes in water until soft. Drain and mash with the milk.
8. Season with salt and pepper to taste.
9. Spoon the mince mixture into a casserole dish.
10. Top with the mash and bake in the oven for 30 minutes until golden brown.

Salmon Fishcakes

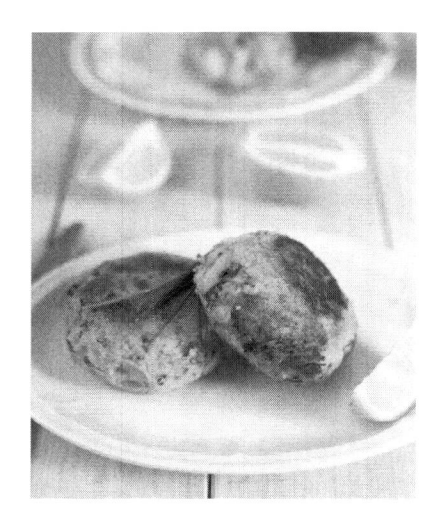

Ingredients

- 400g/14oz (2 cups) skinless salmon fillet, chopped
- 300g/10½oz (1 ¼) cooked broccoli florets, drained well
- 2 lemons, zest only
- 100g/3½oz (1/2 cup) dry white breadcrumbs
- sea salt and freshly ground black pepper
- ½ small bunch fresh parsley, leaves only, finely chopped
- 50g/1¾oz plain flour
- 2 eggs, beaten
- Olive/vegetable oil cooking spray

Method

1. Put the salmon into a food processor along with the cooked broccoli florets and pulse to a finely chopped consistency.
2. Tip into a bowl and add the zest of one lemon.
3. Season with salt and pepper, and mix thoroughly.
4. Divide the mixture into eight equal-sized balls and shape into fish cakes using your hands.
5. Place on a tray lined greaseproof paper and cover with cling film.
6. Leave in the fridge to chill for 20-30 minutes to firm up.
7. Preheat the oven to 220C/425F/Gas 7.
8. Combine the remaining lemon zest with the breadcrumbs, a pinch of salt and pepper and the parsley, and pour into a shallow dish.
9. Prepare a plate of the flour and a shallow dish with the eggs.
10. Coat the fish cakes in flour, shake off any excess and then dip in the beaten eggs.
11. Roll each fishcake in the breadcrumbs until coated on all sides then transfer to a baking tray.
12. Drizzle or spray the fishcakes with a little oil and then bake for 15 minutes, or until golden-brown.
13. Serve with parsley sauce, mushy peas or tinned chopped tomatoes.

Vegetable and Bean Casserole

Ingredients

- 1 onion, peeled and sliced
- 2 carrots, peeled and diced
- 2 parsnips, peeled and diced
- 2 celery stalks, chopped
- 250g, 8oz, 1 cup swede, peeled and diced
- 568ml, 1 pint, 19floz vegetable stock
- 420g, 14oz (1.5 cups) can chopped tomatoes
- 420g, 14oz (1.5 cups) can cannelloni beans, drained
- Low calorie vegetable/olive oil spray

Method

1. Heat non-stick large pan, spray with the oil and add the onion and cook on a medium heat for 5 minutes.
2. Add the other vegetables, cover, and cook over a medium heat for 5 minutes, until they start to soften.
3. Pour in the stock and tinned tomatoes, bring to the boil.
4. Cover and simmer for 10 minutes.
5. Stir in the beans and cook for another 5 minutes, until the vegetables are tender.
6. Serve.

Stage Four—Normal Textured Diet

In the longer term patients will be able to eat a variety of solid textured foods. These recipes can be cooked for all the family and friends. The portion sizes of meals will vary at this stage depending upon the bariatric procedure and the time since the operation. Once the diet is fully established, a tea plate/side plate will be an average sized meal portion. The current recommendations are that half of the plate should be vegetables or salad, a quarter of the plate protein rich foods (meat, fish, soya) and the remaining quarter of the tea plate should be complex carbohydrates such as pasta, rice, potato, couscous, or bread.

Stage Four Recipes

Couscous Salad

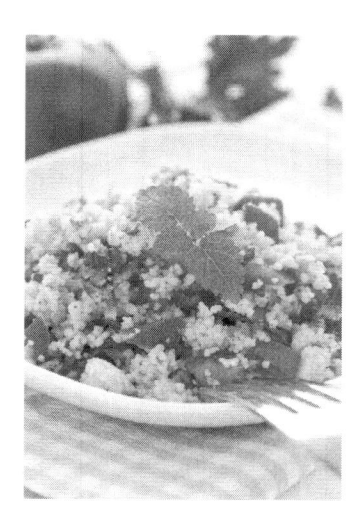

Ingredients

- 100g, 4oz (1/2 cup) couscous
- 200ml, 8 fl. oz vegetable stock
- 2 spring onions
- 1 red pepper
- ½ cucumber
- 50g/2oz (1/4 cup) feta cheese, cubed
- 2 tbsp pesto
- 2 tbsp toasted pine nuts

Method

1. Pour the dried couscous into a large bowl and pour over stock.
2. Cover, then leave for 10 minutes, until fluffy and all the stock has been absorbed.
3. Meanwhile, slice the onions and pepper and dice the cucumber.
4. Add these to the couscous, fork through the pesto, crumble in the feta and then sprinkle over the pine nuts.
5. Serve.

Pasta and Meatballs

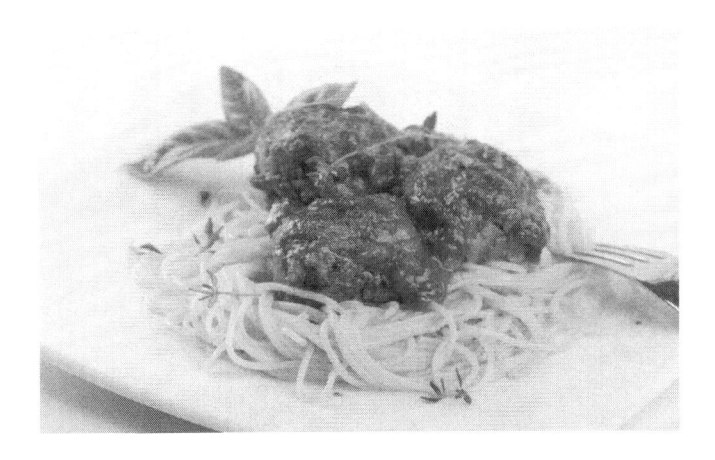

Ingredients

- 150g/5oz onion, finely chopped
- 1 clove garlic, crushed
- 900g/2lb/4 cups lean minced beef

- 2 tbsp freshly chopped herbs such as parsley and rosemary
- 1 egg, beaten
- Salt and freshly ground black pepper
- Low calorie vegetable/olive oil spray

For the tomato sauce

- 110g/4oz onion, finely chopped
- 1 garlic clove, crushed
- 150g/5¼oz reduced fat fresh mozzarella, grated
- Salt and freshly ground black pepper
- 2 x 420g/14oz/1.5 cups canned chopped tomatoes

Method

1. Heat a non-stick saucepan over a gentle heat, spray the olive/vegetable oil and add the onion and garlic.
2. Cover and sweat for four minutes, until soft and a little golden. Allow to cool.
3. In a bowl, mix the minced beef with the cold sweated onion and garlic.
4. Add the herbs and the beaten egg.
5. Season the mixture with salt and pepper.
6. Divide the mixture into approximately 24 round balls.
7. Cover the meatballs and refrigerate until required.
8. Meanwhile, make the tomato sauce. Add a spray of oil then add onion and the crushed garlic to a heated non-stick saucepan, toss until coated, cover, and sweat on a gentle heat until soft and pale golden.

9. Add the canned tomatoes to the onion mixture. Season the contents with salt and freshly ground pepper.
10. Cook the tomato sauce uncovered for approximately 30 minutes.
11. Heat a non-stick saucepan and cook the meatballs for about 10 minutes with the oil spray.
12. When the meatballs are cooked, put them into an ovenproof dish with the tomato sauce and top with the grated reduced fat cheese.
13. Place under a preheated grill until the cheese has melted.
14. Serve with pasta.

Chicken Curry

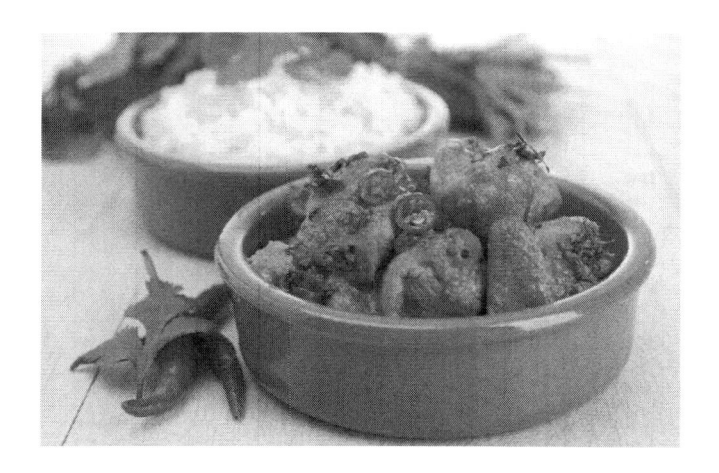

Ingredients

- 1 large onion, finely chopped
- 6 garlic cloves, roughly chopped
- 50g/2oz/1/4 cup ginger, roughly chopped
- 2 tsp cumin seeds
- 1 tsp fennel seed
- 5cm cinnamon stick
- 1 tsp chilli flakes
- 1 tsp garam masala
- 1 tsp turmeric
- 420g/14oz/1.5 cups can chopped tomatoes
- 8 chicken thighs, skinned, boneless
- 250ml chicken stock

- 2 tbsp chopped coriander
- Low calorie vegetable/olive oil spray

Method

1. Add the onion and 3 tablespoons of water to a food processor to make a smooth paste.
2. Put the chopped garlic and ginger into the same food processor and add 4 tablespoons water. Process until smooth and spoon into another small bowl.
3. Heat the spray oil in a non-stick set over a medium heat. Combine the cumin and fennel seeds with the cinnamon and chilli flakes and add to the pan in one go. Swirl everything around for about 30 seconds until the spices release a fragrant aroma.
4. Add the onion paste. Fry until the water evaporates and the onions turn a lovely dark golden - this should take about 7-8 minutes. Add the garlic and ginger paste and cook for another 2 minutes – stirring all the time.
5. Stir in the garam masala, turmeric, and sugar and continue cooking for 20 seconds before tipping in the tomatoes. Continue cooking on a medium heat for about 10 minutes without a lid until the tomatoes reduce and darken.
6. Cut the chicken thighs into 3cm chunks and add to the pan once the tomatoes have thickened to a paste. Cook for 5 minutes to coat the chicken in the masala and seal in the juices, and then pour over the hot chicken stock.
7. Simmer for 8-10 minutes without a lid until the chicken is tender and the masala lightly thickened – you might need to add an extra stock or water.

8. Sprinkle with chopped coriander and serve with flatbread or rice.

For further recipes and meal ideas go to **simply***bariatrics*.com

Chapter 17

Top Tips for after Surgery

After surgery, many patients ask about tips for eating out, buying new clothes, and how to avoid over-eating.

Many more tips can be found on our website at **simply***bariatrics*.com.

Eating Out

Learning how to eat out in a restaurant after surgery can be one of the biggest challenges. Here are some of the hints and tips:

Top Ten Tips for Eating Out

1. Check the restaurant menu online and plan the order before arrival.
2. Choose a starter portion rather than a main course.
3. Order a child's portion for the main meal.
4. Try a sharing platter or tapas with friends and family.
5. Share a meal with someone else.
6. Ask the waiter if leftovers can be taken home.
7. Have a coffee (not a latte) instead of a dessert.
8. If food is left on the plate, cover it with a napkin then the waiter won't ask any questions.
9. Avoid buffets, which encourage eating too much.
10. Try to be the slowest eater.

Buying New Clothes

As weight is lost after surgery, many may find their clothing size changes rapidly, which can make shopping quite expensive. These are some of the suggestions given by our patients to bear in mind during that initial rapid weight-loss phase.

1. Buy clothes and sell clothes in charity shops or online auctions—- these can be very nice and very cheap (and selling clothes that are too big helps fund the purchase of smaller sizes).
2. Have clothing altered
3. Seek out online "clothes swap" sites where bariatric patients trade clothes.
4. Buy and wear belts or scarves that can wrap around skirts, trousers and tops to make them look and fit better—accessorise!
5. Don't throw away all old clothes straight away. Keep at least one piece of clothing as a reminder of how much weight has been lost.

Covering Loose Skin

Loose skin is a common problem after bariatric surgery, and is nothing to be ashamed of. However, there are a number of methods for dressing to cover this up, if desired.

1. Buy some Lycra underwear that are designed to help smooth and pull in the loose skin. Many high street shops stock these items.
2. Buy mid-length sleeves if under-arm skin is a concern. Some tops are very light and attractive, which can be useful in the summer.
3. Wear a sarong or light shawl/scarf on holiday to cover thighs and arms.
4. Darker colours can often be very slimming.
5. Bra size may change dramatically after surgery. It is recommended that it be re-measured—having a well fitting bra will help with your figure.

Avoid Over-Eating

One of the most difficult things about having bariatric surgery is changing lifestyle habits. Patients have described many different ways of avoiding over eating.

The best way to avoid this is to listen to your body. Are feelings of hunger genuine or is your desire to eat from boredom/stress/habit?

1. Have a glass of water 20-30 minutes before a meal. We often feel hungry when we are in fact thirsty.
2. Go for a walk/play with children/phone a friend/pick up a hobby. This can often distract you and is very effective if you are eating out of boredom.
3. Do not buy cakes/biscuits/crisps/chocolate. If they are not in the house, it is much more difficult to eat them!

4. Lock away the 'naughty' foods and give the key to a partner or the children. This is effective if others want them in the house.
5. When the desire for something that shouldn't be eaten is strong, make a point of delaying gratification. Decide that if the item is still wanted later, it can be eaten. Often "later" comes around and the craving is long forgotten!
6. Don't be too strict. Everyone needs a little treat occasionally; just make sure to indulge in moderation. Have a piece of chocolate and give the rest of the bar to a partner/friend. This will prevent eating the whole thing.

Follow Up and Support

Successful weight loss in the long run means it is important to have regular follow up and constant support.

Always have the following information on hand:

1. Date, time, and location of next appointment.
2. Contact details for the dietitian, nurse, and doctor.
3. Contact details of people from the support group.
4. Information on useful websites and forums.

For more of these tips and hints, visit **simply***bariatrics*.com

Chapter 18

Useful Links

Register FREE on www.**simply**bariatrics.com

This book is a product of **Simply**bariatrics, a company designed and run by experts in the field of weight loss surgery. The success of weight loss surgery is determined by proper planning and excellent post-operative care, which are the fundamental principals underlying **Simply**bariatrics.

Our website, www.**simply**bariatrics.com contains revolutionary material from videos, articles, forums and 'Ask the Experts' databases, to our online aftercare programmes. These can support you through your weight loss journey and in the years afterwards.

Here you can find useful tools such as the Relationship with Food Diary in Chapter 14, a food and symptom diary, which can help track your progress, more recipes, tips, and hints for exercise.

To get a copy of a table comparing different weight loss surgeries please email us at hello@simplybariatrics.com

Find us on Twitter and Facebook!

Other useful links:

www.bomss.org.uk	British Obesity and Metabolic Surgery Society
www.asmbs.org	American Society of Metabolic and Bariatric Surgery
www.ifso.com	International Federation for the Surgery of Obesity and Metabolic Disorders
www.ossanz.com.au	Obesity Surgery Society of Australia and New Zealand

Printed in Great Britain
by Amazon